EAST RENFREWSHIRE
1003158 8

KT-167-116

OVID-19

t you need to know about the

RONAVIRUS

d the race for the vaccine

COVID-19

What you need to know about the CORONAVIRUS and the race for the vaccine

DR MICHAEL MOSLEY

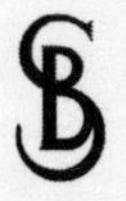

The content of this book is intended to inform, entertain and provoke your thinking. This is not intended as medical advice. It may, however, make you question current medical and nutritional advice. That's your choice. It's your life and health in your hands. Neither the author nor the publisher can be held responsible or liable for any loss or claim arising from the use, or misuse, of the content of this book.

If you have underlying health problems or any specific health needs that may require medical supervision, or have any doubts about the information contained in this book, you should contact a qualified medical, dietary, or other appropriate professional, especially before embarking upon any dietary, weight loss or fitness regime.

Published in 2020 by Short Books
Unit 316, ScreenWorks, 22 Highbury Grove,
London, N5 2ER

10 9 8 7 6 5 4 3 2 1

Copyright © Parenting Matters Ltd, 2020

Michael Mosley has asserted his right under the Copyright, Designs and Patents Act 1988 to be identified as the author of this work. All rights reserved. No part of this publication may be reproduced, stored in a retrieval system or transmitted in any form, or by any means (electronic, mechanical, or otherwise) without the prior written permission of both the copyright owners and the publisher.

A CIP catalogue record for this book is
available from the British Library.

ISBN: 978-1-78072-461-4

Printed at CPI Group (UK) Ltd, Croydon, CR0 4YY

MIX
Paper from
responsible sources
FSC
www.fsc.org
FSC® C0204

Illustrations by E.K. Mosley
Cover design by Smith & Gilmour
Cover image © EZME
Cover text and design © Short Books Ltd

EAST RENFREWSHIRE COUNCIL
1003158 8
Askews & Holts
17-Mar-2021
614.592
EA

CONTENTS

Introduction

Chapter 1: Portrait of a serial killer

Chapter 2: How the virus escaped

Chapter 3: Questions and answers

Chapter 4: How to bolster your immunity

Chapter 5: The race for a vaccine

Chapter 6: The future

Introduction

Few of us have lived through anything like this or had to face such an uncertain future. As I watched fireworks explode on New Year's Eve, I was completely unaware that earlier that day the Chinese had announced the outbreak of a novel virus in the city of Wuhan. Nor would I have been particularly concerned.

As a science journalist I have, down the years, made a number of documentaries about the dangers of microbes jumping from animals to humans and creating a devastating worldwide pandemic. I have also written articles about how vulnerable we are to the emergence of a sly new pathogen. But in my heart of hearts I never thought it would be as bad as this. I assumed, as so many others did, that when a new, infectious agent appeared we would be able to use the high tech tools at our disposal to isolate and stamp it out.

Yet the world had plenty of warnings that an unstoppable pandemic was not only possible but highly likely. In the 40 years since I went to medical school there have been numerous outbreaks of novel infectious diseases caused by viruses going from animals to humans, ranging from AIDS to bird flu, swine flu, SARS, MERS and Ebola. AIDS alone has killed over 30 million people and continues to kill another 700,000 every year.

What should have worried governments is that over recent decades the number of fresh outbreaks has been growing, with new ones emerging at four times the rate that they were back in the 1980s. The World Health Organisation has pointed out again and again that it was only a matter of time before something like this happened.

And now it is here. Amongst us. A terrifying science fiction story which has suddenly become real. And our best hope, indeed our only hope of bringing this virus under control, now lies with the scientists. We need their computer models, their ability to create effective treatment and, above all, we need them to create a safe and effective vaccine.

This book is about the race to create that vaccine. It is also a distillation of what we currently know about SARS-CoV-2, how it spreads and how you can best protect yourself from being struck down. I will answer some of the most common queries that come my way, and end by taking a peek into the future, speculating what it will look like.

I have been fortunate enough to gain access to numerous experts who have been generous with their time. I have relied on their expertise, as well as the extraordinary amount of excellent news coverage produced by my fellow science journalists from around the world. I have also tried, to the best of my ability, to keep up with the huge number of new studies which have poured out of science journals over the months that I have been writing this book.

No one knows how bad this pandemic will become or how long it will last. I am guardedly optimistic that science will come to our rescue and that we will develop more accurate tests and more effective treatments – as well as that all important vaccine. I am also optimistic that this will be the wake-up call we need to combat future, even more lethal microbial threats.

1 Portrait of a serial killer

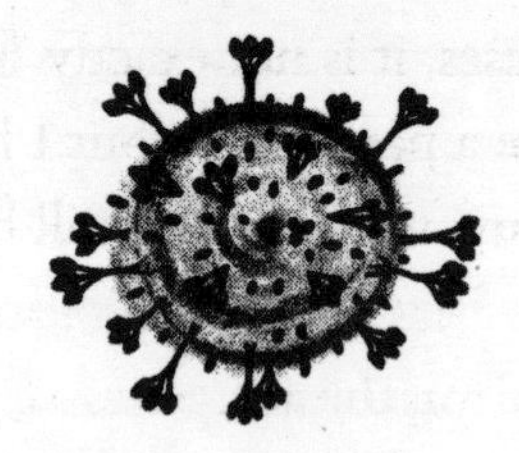

The Chinese military strategist, Sun Tzu, wrote in his classic book *The Art of War* that victory comes from understanding your enemy. So what have we learnt about this novel virus?

We know that SARS-CoV-2, or Severe Acute Respiratory Syndrome Coronavirus 2, to give it its full name, is tiny, just 120 nanometres (billionths of a metre) across. You could fit a hundred million viral particles on the head of a pin and yet you would only need to be exposed to a few hundred to get infected. If you do get infected and develop symptoms then the disease you get is called "Covid-19".

SARS-CoV-2 is a killer with a range of impressive superpowers, including the ability to travel amongst us, undetected, infect almost everyone it meets and then reproduce liberally, before jumping off in search of a new host. It has found a range of ingenious ways to hide from its most deadly enemy (our immune system) and thanks to the airplane, can travel from one side of the globe to the other at astonishing speed.

Like other viruses, it is not exactly "alive", and it certainly doesn't have a personality, but I like to think of it as a cunning enemy; that is why I will be using the metaphors of war when it comes to the battle that we face.

It is also why, for the purposes of this narrative, I am going to give the virus agency and purpose, which it clearly doesn't have. Viruses don't plan, seek out or attempt to avoid. They are mindless scraps of genetic material, brilliantly adapted by evolution for one purpose: to reproduce and spread as far and as fast as they can.

And finally, although its proper name is SARS-CoV-2, from now on, for simplicity's sake, I am going to refer to it as the Covid-19 virus.

The Covid-19 virus represents the greatest public health crisis of the last hundred years. As we'll see, only by mobilising the scientific community and by committing huge resources are we likely to be able to keep the death toll down and return to any sort of normality.

Meet the enemy

Despite the huge threat it poses, the Covid-19 virus is relatively simple. Its core is a single strand of Ribonucleic acid (RNA), which stores all the genetic information the virus needs to reproduce. Think of it as a Covid-making instruction manual, just 30,000 letters long.

A human-building instruction manual, by comparison, comes in the form of DNA, which is tightly packed into our cells in 46 "manuals", known as chromosomes. Put those 46 manuals together and you get our genome, which consists of 6.4 billion letters. If you took all the DNA from just one of our cells and stretched it out (I've done it), then it would be around 2 metres long. Take it out of all of your cells and it would be 10 billion miles long. We are large, complicated and clever. Covid-19 is not. Yet it has us on the run.

This short strand of Covid-19 RNA is protected by a fatty outer membrane, which is quite fragile. It breaks apart when it meets soap and water, which is why hand-washing, with soap, is so important.

The outer membrane of the virus is studded with club-like spikes which give the virus its name (corona, meaning "crowns") and which it uses to get into our cells. These are also a potential area of vulnerability as it is those spikes, as we will see in chapter 5, that most vaccine makers are targeting.

The way the virus spreads is mainly through coughs and sneezes. If someone who is currently infected with the virus coughs or sneezes near you, out will come a cloud of viruses. If you are unlucky enough to inhale just a few hundred particles, then they could get into your throat and will immediately start "looking" for cells to invade.

The invasion begins

The good news is that your body has evolved numerous defences to protect you against just such a threat. The bad news is that your body has a fatal flaw. On the surface of many of your cells there is an enzyme called ACE2.

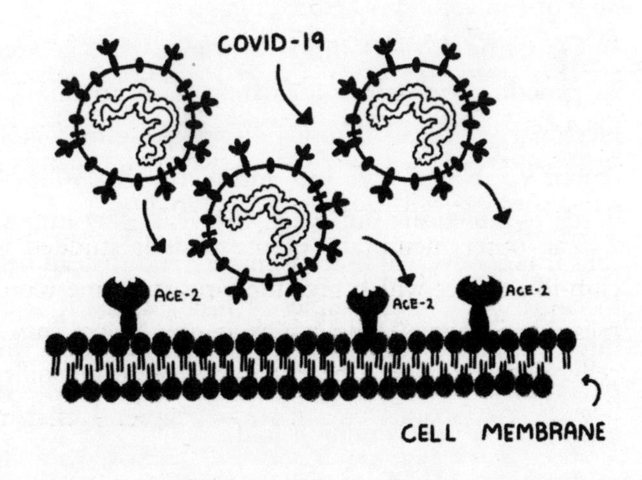

These ACE2 enzymes play an important role in controlling your blood pressure. In fact some of the most popular drugs used to control blood pressure are called ACE inhibitors. They do this by binding ACE2 enzymes on the surface of blood vessels, which causes them to relax, lowering your blood pressure.

We don't know how it happened, but the spikes on the surface of the Covid-19 virus are just the right shape to lock onto these ACE2 enzymes and bind tightly. Once that occurs it is like inserting a key into a lock and turning. The human cell opens up and the virus slips in.

ACE-2 enzymes are found throughout your body, including your throat, lungs, eyes and the inside of your nose. That is why you should wash your hands whenever you have been outside and resist the urge to touch your nose or rub your eyes before doing so.

Once the virus is inside a human cell, it releases its genetic code and immediately starts to hijack the machinery of the cell. Your cells are like mini factories, geared up to make the bits and pieces that your body needs to function. But when the virus gets into your cells it takes over all that machinery and instead begins to churn out endless copies of itself, which it releases into your body, ready to infect more cells. It does this at phenomenal speed. With each day that passes the virus can multiply itself a million-fold.

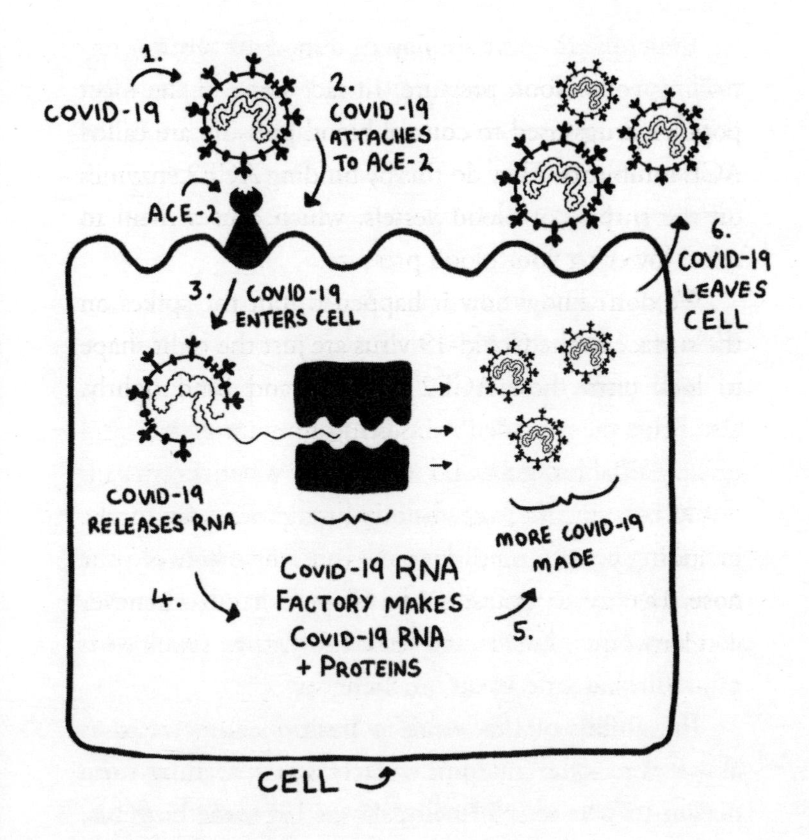

Evading detection

When any virus gets into your body and starts multiplying, your immune system should swiftly spring into action and unleash hell. But the Covid-19 virus has lots of tricks up its sleeve to help it evade detection.

For starters, when your cells are invaded by a foreign microbe they are supposed to send out distress signals, warning your body that it is being attacked. But the Covid-19 virus can do the equivalent of cutting the telephone lines, silencing the alarms before they go off. That way it can hide from your defence system while it continues to multiply.

Another trick the virus uses is to cover the spikes that stick out of its surface with sugars, known as glycans. These disguise the fact that they are viral proteins which also helps them evade the body's immune system.

It is all about getting a head start. What the virus is doing is trying to overwhelm your defences by means of a fast, silent, powerful attack. It is a race between the virus's ability to multiply and your ability to respond. The outcome of that race dictates whether you have a mild illness or end up in intensive care.

The ability of this virus to multiply undetected is also key to its extraordinary success at spreading from person to person. Normally, if you get something like the flu, within a couple of days you will develop a cough or fever. That is a sign that your body has been attacked and your immune system is trying to fight back. It is also a very useful warning to you that you should go to bed and self-isolate, and to other people that they need to steer clear of you.

Because the Covid-19 virus is able to silence the

alarms, when someone is infected it typically takes them around five days to start showing symptoms, and some people never do. They become what is known as "asymptomatic carriers". They continue with their daily lives blissfully unaware that they are now shedding potentially lethal viruses everywhere they go.

The story of Typhoid Mary

One of the most famous examples of an asymptomatic carrier was a woman who became known as "Typhoid Mary".

Typhoid fever is caused by a salmonella infection. Worldwide it kills at least 14,000 people every year, many of them children. It used to be a major killer in crowded cities, like London, but by the beginning of the 20th century better sanitation meant there were fewer outbreaks in affluent countries.

In 1907 there was a particularly nasty outbreak in New York City. One of the families who had been affected hired a researcher called George Soper to find out what had happened. He eventually discovered that an Irish woman called Mary Mallon had worked in many of the houses where people had subsequently got typhoid.

Objecting strongly, Mary was taken to a hospital and tested. Although she was completely healthy, when they tested her poo they discovered lots of salmonella bacteria. Mary was an asymptomatic carrier and in a time before antibiotics there was nothing they could do to cure her. To protect the general public she was put into isolation.

She was confined to a hospital bungalow for three years and then released on condition that she never worked as a cook again. But she just changed her name and went on working, spreading typhoid wherever she went. She was finally caught, a few years later, while cooking in a hospital where an outbreak of typhoid led to 25 people becoming infected and two dying. Mary (now nicknamed "Typhoid Mary") was arrested and kept in confinement until her death, 23 years later.

The Munich Cluster

We first learnt about the importance of asymptomatic carriers of Covid-19 thanks to some very smart detective work done in Germany.[1]

In late January a woman from Shanghai visited a company, based near Munich, that makes car parts. She felt a bit ill while she was there, but assumed that was because she was jet lagged. She stayed for a few days in Munich and then flew home. On her return to Shanghai, still feeling ill, she went to see her doctor, was tested and found to be positive for Covid-19.

When, soon afterwards, a middle-aged man from the German auto company went down with a mild, flu-like illness, he was isolated and tested. He had Covid-19. The Germans swiftly traced and found eight others from the company who were now infected, and brought them into München Klinik Schwabing hospital to be monitored and treated.

At this point very little was known about the virus or how it spreads. What the scientists discovered, after interviewing their new patients, was really disturbing. One man had got infected after being in a room where someone else had sneezed. Another had got it from a brief handshake.

Colonel Roman Wolfel, Director of the Bundeswehr Institute of Microbiology, told me that throat swabs taken from "the Munich cluster" revealed that not only were their throats infected, but that they had begun to shed lots of viruses soon after being infected. As he explained, this was worrying.

"A high viral load in the throat at the very onset of symptoms suggests that individuals with Covid-19 are infectious very early on, in some cases before they are even aware of being ill."

The researchers also discovered that being infected could lead to a range of different outcomes. While one of the older patients developed pneumonia, another had no symptoms at all. Most had dry coughs, but only two of them developed a fever. Four of the nine lost all sense of smell, which was probably due to the virus infecting nerve cells in their noses.

The good news was that most of the patients started making antibodies against the virus after six days, and by 12 days they had all done so. Once the antibody levels rose, the rate of viral shedding fell, fast. Colonel Wolfel said that they intend to follow this group of patients to see what happens to their antibody levels over time.

This type of research will play an important role in the development of a vaccine, as I will describe in chapter 5.

Why were the Germans so well prepared for the outbreak? "Because we realised that such an event could happen at any time and we had invested in the equipment and expertise needed to respond," was Colonel Wolfel's matter-of-fact reply.

Why is Covid-19 so much worse than other coronaviruses?

This ability to infect someone else before you yourself have major symptoms is one of the key differences between the Covid-19 virus, and its close relative, SARS-CoV, the coronavirus that caused an outbreak of a respiratory disease called SARS, nearly 20 years ago.

SARS began as an outbreak in China in 2002. It hit the headlines when an American businessman travelling from China to Singapore via Vietnam began to show signs of a pneumonia-like illness during the flight. He was taken off the plane in Vietnam and later died in a hospital in Hanoi. Several of the medical staff who looked after him later developed symptoms and one of them died.

SARS soon spread to other countries, including Hong Kong, Taiwan and Singapore. It was much more lethal than Covid-19, killing nearly 10% of those who got infected. But the good thing about SARS is that people didn't start becoming infectious until they were already showing symptoms of the disease. Which meant that that particular coronavirus wasn't able to hide amongst us.

The SARS virus was also not as good at binding to the ACE2 enzymes in our respiratory tract as the Covid-19 virus which made it far less infectious.

And because the SARS virus did not have those two superpowers, the ability to hide and the ability to bind, it never turned into a pandemic. Although SARS caused a panic at the time, there were just 8000 reported cases of it and "only" 774 people died. Then it fizzled out. There have been no new cases of SARS since 2004.

The flying virus

The fact that the Covid-19 virus can be carried by people who have few, if any, symptoms meant, in the early days, it could fly around the world with great ease.

One of my sons, Dan, is a good example of how easily the virus can jump continents. Until March 2020, Dan was living in Melbourne, Australia, with a couple of doctors. When countries all over the world began closing their borders because of the virus, he decided it was time to get on a plane home.

He left Melbourne on Saturday 21st March and arrived at Heathrow airport on Sunday 22nd. I picked him up from the airport and brought him home. He was cheerful and appeared perfectly healthy. We were delighted to see him back.

The following morning Dan got a call from one of his former flatmates to say that he had developed a cough over the weekend and had just been tested positive for Covid-19.

The next day, Tuesday 24th March, Dan also started to develop classic signs of Covid-19, including a dry cough, fever, muscle ache and a headache. He was ill for a couple of days and then swiftly recovered, apart from his sense of smell, which took many weeks to return.

Although he didn't know it at the time, Dan was

almost certainly shedding viruses when he went to the airport in Melbourne and when he got on the plane. He wore a mask while he was flying but he could still have given it to other passengers.

Since he had to change planes in Thailand, he could also have infected people at Bangkok airport. If he had had SARS he would have been so obviously ill that he would not have been able to travel. He and his viruses would have remained in Melbourne.

Where did the Covid-19 virus come from?

Although we describe it as a "new" virus, the Covid-19 virus has almost certainly been around, in a slightly different form, for a very long time.

Recent studies suggest that the ancestor of this particular virus has been living in horseshoe bats in southern China for thousands of years and that the bats have evolved to the point that they were no longer bothered by it.

But it seems that the Covid-19 virus, like HIV, Ebola and the SARS virus, was not content just to infect one species of animal. It bided its time.

The first warnings that there were some potentially very dangerous pathogens living in the bat caves of China came in 2013, when scientists working at the

Wuhan Institute of Virology reported that they had isolated a coronavirus from horseshoe bats which could infect human cells.

Researchers from Harvard Medical School, who later studied this same coronavirus in the lab, found it was especially good at infecting cells grown from the human respiratory tract. The Harvard scientists warned that this particular coronavirus was "poised for human emergence". They were concerned that it might jump from the bats and start infecting humans at any time.

They were right. We now know that the virus which the Harvard team were so worried about in 2016 is 96% identical to the Covid-19 virus that is spreading amongst us now. The tragedy is that no one in authority paid any attention to these warnings.

The reason that the Harvard scientists were so concerned about this particular virus is because bats have been the source of a couple of other very significant coronavirus outbreaks, in particular SARS and MERS (Middle East Respiratory Syndrome).

SARS, as I've just explained, erupted in 2002, killed 774 people and then disappeared. MERS, which began in Saudi Arabia in 2012 and spread to 20 countries, is more lethal than SARS, killing 1 in 3 of those who get it. But like SARS it never really took off. It is still out there, and there are occasional outbreaks, but when it does get into the human population it only manages to kill a few people before it is isolated and contained.

Why do coronaviruses which are harmless to bats seem to be so dangerous to us (or at least to some of us)? Because bats are really good at handling viral infections. When a bat gets infected by a virus, it mounts a particularly rapid and fierce immune response. This means that any viruses that have managed to get a foothold in a bat's body can only survive if they "learn" how to reproduce quickly in a very hostile environment. So when, the Covid-19 virus jumped from bats to another animal species it was already battle-hardened.

We don't know exactly when that jump happened or which animal it first jumped into. It may have been a human, or it may have been another animal.

We know that SARS came from bats and reached humans via the Asian palm civet, a mongoose-like mammal which is eaten in some parts of southern China. Research has shown that palm civets were sold in food markets linked to the SARS outbreak, and samples taken from civets sold in those markets have shown they are riddled with SARS virus.

MERS, which also originated in bats, came to us via camels. They are still a source of infection.

Although we don't know for certain which animal, if any, acted as an intermediary for Covid-19, the likeliest candidate is a creature called the pangolin – a scaly, ant-eating animal which is killed and sold in large numbers for its scales, which are still heavily used in Chinese traditional medicine. One good thing that may come out of this disaster is that the Chinese authorities might finally stamp down on the sale of these and other highly endangered species. Fingers crossed.

Whatever its origins, Covid-19 is like a monstrous mutant hybrid of other coronaviruses that have come before. It can infect us without our knowing. And it spreads easily and silently.

How the virus spreads

Let's take a look, in a bit more detail, at how this particular virus spreads. Imagine you are in a supermarket and someone in a nearby aisle, who is unknowingly infected, coughs or sneezes. Viruses don't travel naked, they travel in droplets of fluid. A single cough can produce around 3,000 droplets, which travel from your mouth at almost 50mph and release at least 200,000,000 (two hundred million) virus particles into the air. Some of those droplets, the heavier ones, will fall on the floor or onto nearby shelves of food.[2]

If you are more than 2 metres (6 feet) away from someone who is coughing there is a good chance that

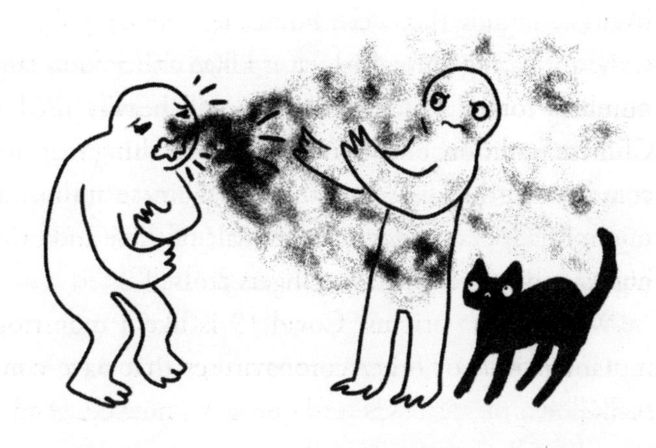

you will avoid contact with these the big droplets while they are in the air. That's why social distancing is so important. But the really small droplets, known as "aerosols", can, according to a study by the National Institutes of Health, remain suspended in the air, like cigarette smoke, for up to three hours.[3]

An example of how potent aerosols can be was a choir rehearsal in America which ended in tragedy. In early March 2020, 60 singers of the Skagit Valley Chorale turned up at Mount Vernon Presbyterian Church for their regular practice. Although they knew there was a threat from Covid-19, nobody appeared to be ill and the choir took what felt like suitable precautions. They all used hand sanitisers and they avoided handshakes or close physical contact. After a couple of hours of singing they went home.

Three weeks later, 45 of them had either been diagnosed or come down with symptoms of Covid-19. Two of them had died. No one really knows what happened that evening but it is likely that someone who was an asymptomatic carrier produced a fine cloud of viral particles while singing heartily, enough to infect people nearby.

Going back to the example of the supermarket. As you walk down the aisle where someone has just coughed, it is possible that you will inhale viral particles. Or perhaps you will pick up viruses on your hands from the droplets that have fallen on the food that you are about to buy. Or you may get them from the trolley handle. Before you get to the check out, and without thinking, you rub your eye or touch the inside of your nose.

The virus is in.

What the virus does when it gets inside your body

When it gets into your body, the first area that the virus is likely to infect is the cells that line your nose and your upper throat. So one of your first symptoms is likely to be a dry, persistent cough.

Some virus particles will fly past the throat and

travel down into your gut, where they latch onto ACE2 enzymes in your intestines and may cause diarrhoea.

Much more dangerous is if the virus particles go down your windpipe and into your lungs. Your lungs are filled with ACE2 enzymes, making them a wonderful breeding ground for this virus. Once the virus is in your lungs you will start to develop symptoms of pneumonia. These, over time, may include a cough, fever, sweating, shaking, chills, shortness of breath and a stabbing chest pain. As we'll see, these symptoms are caused, not just by the virus, but by your body's attempt to fight the virus off.

So what happens next?

Days 1 to 2

Let's assume the virus starts by just infecting your throat. For the next couple of days it multiplies rapidly, jumping eagerly from cell to cell, turning each one of them into a virus-producing factory. And all the while you feel absolutely fine, completely unaware of the looming threat.

Day 3

By day 3 of the infection you are shedding so many viruses that you can infect someone else by shaking their hands or simply sitting at the same table in a work canteen. If you are eating with someone who has eaten garlic, and you can smell it, then you are close enough to get infected.

Before there was a worldwide lockdown, you might have hopped on a plane at this point to another part of the world, gone to a big football match or taken part in the Mardi Gras in New Orleans. And all the while you would have been shedding viruses every time you talked, coughed or sneezed.

Although the virus has done all it can to evade your immune system, at some point your body will realise that something is seriously wrong.

Your innate defences

Your body's first line of defence is known as the innate immune system. It consists of cells that are always patrolling, always on the alert for an invader. We know this is a very ancient system, in evolutionary terms, because it is also found in plants and insects.

One of the first things the innate system does, when it senses an invader, is release proteins called interferons. They get their name because they interfere with the virus's ability to replicate and spread. As well as trying to stop the virus reproducing, the interferons recruit other parts of your immune system, such as neutrophils, to try and destroy the invaders.

Neutrophils are a type of white blood cell. When

they are alerted, they head for the infection, determined to neutralise the enemy. They are most effective against bacteria and fungi, which they either phagocytose ("eat") or try to poison. Against viral infections they are something of a double-edged sword. They start off by trying to destroy the viral invaders, but can end up being part of a catastrophic battle inside your body, called a cytokine storm (see page 36).

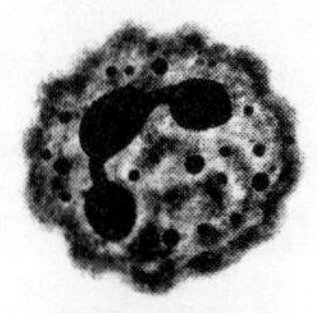

A NEUTROPHIL

Another of the cells of the innate system that soon gets involved in tackling viral infections are macrophages. They are one of the great watchdogs of the immune system, scavengers whose job is to roam around and eat anything they come across that looks suspicious (macrophage means "big eater"). Later, if the job is too big to handle, they too will call on other parts of your immune system to help.

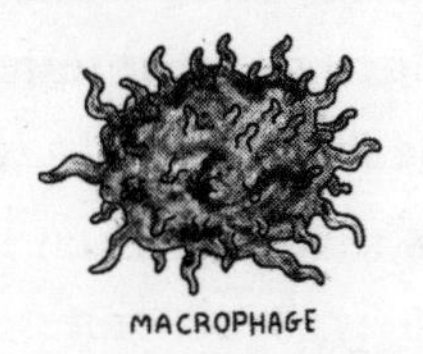

MACROPHAGE

If you are young and healthy, there is a chance that the innate part of your immune system will be able to keep the virus under control until the big guns arrive. You may get a mild cough, a bit of a temperature, or nothing at all.

Day 5

When my son Dan, who is 25 years old, got Covid-19, he developed most of the classic symptoms (cough, fever and aching muscles), yet he was never especially ill and within a few days he was completely fine.

If you are not so lucky, what happens next is that the virus travels from your throat down into your lungs. Your dry cough just gets worse and worse. You find it hard to breathe, develop a fever (typically over 38°C) and start to feel real bone ache. Most people, particularly if they have someone to look after them, try to ride this out. They take paracetamol, drink plenty of water and hope their immune system will come to their rescue.

The adaptive response

The next stage in the battle with the virus involves the so-called "adaptive" part of your immune system. Here we see the activation of T-killer cells, whose job is to seek out and destroy cells that have been infected and taken over by Covid-19.

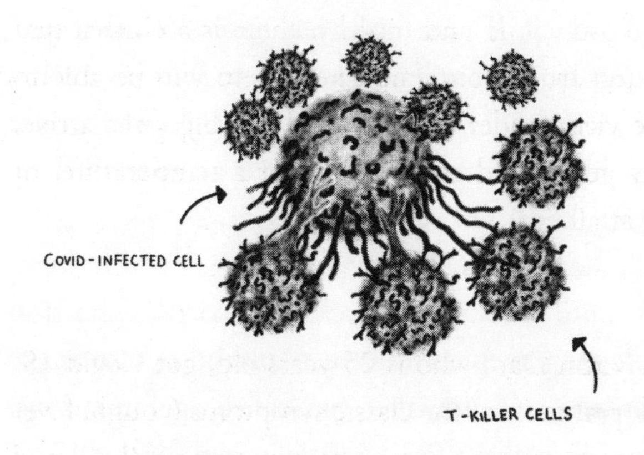

The adaptive response also involves the release of billions of antibodies by plasma B cells, which try to incapacitate or destroy any viruses that are on the loose:

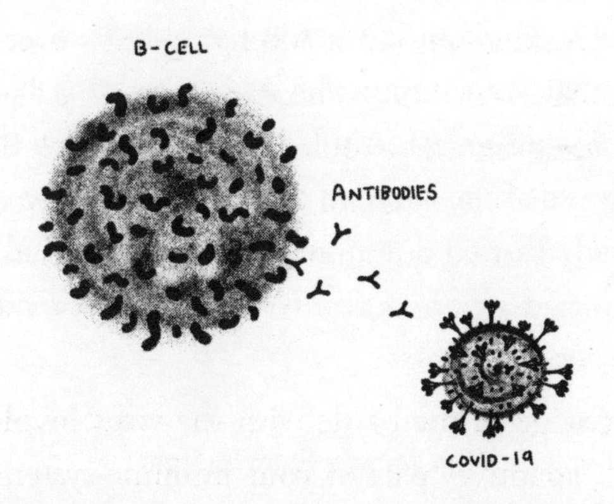

These Y-shaped antibodies have to be exactly the right shape to target a particular virus, in this case the one that causes Covid-19. If your body has never seen that particular virus before it will take a while to start producing and cranking out the right-shaped, targeted antibodies. It is a bit like a factory having to tool up to make new parts at very short notice.

Antibodies do lots of different things. We have "neutralising" antibodies which latch on to viruses and stop them infecting even more cells. Antibodies also make virus particles stick together (it's called agglutination), which in turn makes them an easier target for the rest of the immune system.

On top of that, antibodies activate hungry white cells, which come along and attack anything the antibody has latched onto.

Rising levels of antibodies in the blood is a good sign – a sign that your immune system is fighting back, but it can come quite late in this illness. We know this, not only because of the Munich cluster, but because of a rigorous study carried out at an Australian hospital, where they admitted a woman from Wuhan with Covid-19.

The Woman From Wuhan

The story begins in February 2020 when a 47-year-old Chinese woman went to the emergency department of a hospital in Melbourne. She had flown in from Wuhan 11 days earlier and had developed a cough about a week after arriving. So, for at least a week she had been travelling around Melbourne, shedding viruses and infecting others.

When she arrived at the hospital she complained of a sore throat, a dry cough and chest pain. The medical staff examined her and found that she was short of breath and had a high temperature. A nasal swab revealed that she had Covid-19.

They took daily swabs and blood samples throughout her stay in the hospital.

Even though she had had symptoms for more than a week, her immune system had yet to show signs of mounting a full response. It was only after she had been in hospital for three days that her doctors detected a significant rise in her antibody levels. At that point her body also started churning out lots more T-killer cells, whose job is to latch on to infected cells and destroy them.

Once her immune system got going, it was incredibly effective. With minimal medical support her body got on top of the Covid-19 virus. Within 11 days of admission she was discharged.

So you can see that a healthy and active immune system is critical to fighting off the virus. Which could explain why older people are so much more vulnerable than the young. People like me, who are over 60, tend to have weaker, less efficient immune systems and, initially, may be slower to mount an adequate response. Paradoxically, later in the illness older people's immune systems are prone to overreact, creating a surge of aggressive immune cells that can damage the lungs and other organs.

Days 9 to 11

Nine days after being infected most people will either have recovered or, like the woman from Wuhan, find that their symptoms have started to get much worse. If you start becoming increasingly breathless you will almost certainly need to go to hospital to be tested for the virus, and treated. The medical team there will take bloods, listen to your breathing and you may also need a CT scan of your lungs. What they will be looking for are "ground-glass opacities", fuzzy spots in your lungs caused by fluid. These are a sign that you may have started to develop a very nasty form of pneumonia called acute-respiratory-distress syndrome, or ARDS. That's because the alveoli, the tiny air sacs in your lungs, are filling with fluid, reducing your ability to absorb oxygen.

When the virus infects your alveoli, your immune system responds by flooding the area with the heavy guns, including T-killer cells, antibodies and cytokines. But this can be the beginning of what is called a "cytokine storm", whereby, in its eagerness to destroy the virus, your body's own immune system starts destroying healthy tissue as well. It is like having a battle in the middle of a city full of civilians. There is going to be enormous collateral damage.

Once your alveoli, or air sacs, become damaged and fill with fluid, you can't get enough oxygen into your body to keep your brain and other organs properly supplied.

At this point, you may well get sent to intensive care, where you will be looked after by nurses and doctors fully garbed with PPE, who may appear rather frightening. But by now you will probably be gasping for air, unconcerned about your surroundings.

The medical staff will have to swiftly decide whether you are given extra oxygen via a mask or whether you should be intubated, sedated and go on a ventilator. Being intubated involves having a tube passed down your throat and into your lungs. You will be relying on a ventilator to keep you alive. This is done as a last resort. Once you need to be ventilated the chances of dying are high. Even if you survive there tend to be long term consequences to health.

By this point the battle between your immune system and the virus isn't confined to your lungs. It will have spread far and wide, through your blood. The liver, kidneys, guts and brain all come under attack. You may also get increased blood clotting, and inflammation in the heart, which is why anyone with pre-existing heart disease or high blood pressure is so much more vulnerable. Once the virus affects your brain it can also cause seizures.

What the medics are desperately trying to prevent is total organ failure. Under attack from the virus and cut off from a healthy supply of oxygen, organs like the kidneys start to collapse. Sadly, when that happens, there may be little more that can be done. It typically takes three to four weeks to go from infection to death.

How deadly is the new virus?

To estimate how dangerous a virus is, scientists talk about a Case Fatality Rate or CFR. This is calculated by taking the number of people who are known to have the disease and dividing it by the number who die of the disease.

These rates tend to be much higher than what is really happening because it does not include people who have been infected but have no symptoms, or those who have been ill but are never tested.

So you have to take CFR figures with a very large pinch of salt. They are the best we currently have, but the real figures for how deadly the virus is (the Infection Fatality Rate) are likely to be many times lower.

Based on what happened in China, for example, the virus has an overall CFR of 2.3%. But in reality it probably kills less than 0.7%. Which makes it seven times deadlier than flu, but not as deadly as originally feared, and only really dangerous if you are over 60 or have a pre-existing health condition.

Who gets ill from it

Because Covid-19 can be caught from someone else coughing or sneezing, it has been compared to the flu, but it is actually very different, particularly in who it kills.

The great 1918 flu outbreak, known as Spanish flu, infected 500 million people – about a third of the world's population – and killed around 50 million, making it one of the deadliest pandemics in history. But it killed mainly *young* adults. In the US, 99% of those who died were under the age of 65, and mostly between 20 and 40. The worst affected were pregnant women, where death rates were up to 70%. No one knows why.

More recent flu epidemics have been very different, killing mainly the old and the very young. It is adults over the age of 65 and children under the age of five who are at the greatest risk of developing severe complications from the flu, being hospitalised, and dying.

You don't see this with Covid-19. In fact, unless you have a pre-existing condition, the odds of dying from Covid-19 if you are under 30 are less than 1000 to one.

Young children seem to be protected from the worst effects of this virus. Not only do they rarely get symptoms, but they don't seem to readily spread it to adults. A striking example of this was the case of a nine-year-old British boy who got Covid-19 while skiing in the Alps. He had very mild symptoms and returned to school soon afterwards. Despite close contact he did not transmit the Covid virus to his siblings or any of the 100 other people who he came in close contact with before he was diagnosed.

In fact, according to a recent review of the data, there appear to be few documented cases of a child passing Covid-19 to an adult. It is more likely to be the other way round.[4]

Men v women

Kids may not get it badly, but men certainly do. Men, at every age, who get Covid-19 are far more likely to die than women. These figures are taken from the outbreak in Italy, but they are similar to what happened elsewhere:

Age	Women CFR (%)	Men CFR (%)
30-39	0.26	0.43
40-49	0.55	0.91
50-59	1.23	2.05
60-69	4.02	6.67
70-79	11.86	19.7
80-89	17.94	29.9
>=90	19.41	32.3

Remember, case fatality rates represent the percentage of those who went to hospital and tested positive for Covid-19. Since most people have mild symptoms and are never tested, these figures are much higher than the true risk.[5]

Why Covid-19 is so much more dangerous if you are male

There are a couple of theories as to why men are so much more likely to get sick and die from Covid-19 than women.

Firstly women have a more powerful immune system, thanks to the fact that they have two X chromosomes, whereas men only have one. A number of important immune genes are only found on the X chromosome.

A downside to having a more powerful immune system is that women are also more likely to develop auto-immune disease, where the body attacks itself. Examples of auto-immune conditions which are commoner in women include rheumatoid arthritis and multiple sclerosis.

Female hormones may also be protective. To test this claim, in April, doctors at Stony Brook hospital in New York began a study where they gave male and female Covid-19 patients over the age of 55 oestrogen patches, to see if they help. In Los Angeles, they have also recently begun a trial where they give patients a second female hormone, progesterone, which has anti-inflammatory properties.[6]

Another reason why men are so much more likely to get severe Covid-19 is that men tend to have higher rates of obesity, high blood pressure, diabetes, heart disease and lung disease, all of which put you at greater risk of becoming ill and dying from the virus (see chapter 4).

Why does Covid-19 kill mainly older people?

As with men, one of the reasons why older people are so vulnerable is because they are much more likely to have high blood pressure, high blood sugars or high blood fats. Or all three. This is known as metabolic syndrome and the incidence rises with age. Around 30% of adults over the age of 50 in the UK, US and Australia have metabolic syndrome.

According to the science journal *Nature*, people with metabolic syndrome are significantly more likely to die, if they get infected, than people who are healthy. I will be going into this in greater detail in chapter 4.

Older people are also more vulnerable to having a cytokine storm, where the immune system overreacts and starts destroying not just the virus but your heart and lungs as well (see page 36).

Is Covid-19 more dangerous if you come from a particular ethnic group?

One of my sons, Jack, who is a doctor working in an Intensive Care Unit, says it is striking how many of the patients he sees are from black and minority ethnic (BAME) backgrounds. And this is certainly reflected in the data.

The UK's Intensive Care National Audit and Research Centre keeps a record of the ethnicity of patients who end up in intensive care, many of whom then die. Below is a comparison between intensive care patients in an average flu year and Covid-19.[7]

	Covid-19	Flu (2017- 2019)
Average age	59 years	58 years
White	66%	88%
Mixed	2%	1%
Asian	15%	6%
Black	11%	3%
Other	6%	2%

What is striking is that while the percentage of white, black and Asian patients who end up on intensive care during a flu epidemic reflect their percentages in the UK population, things are very different when it comes to Covid-19.

If you come from a black or Asian ethnic background you are much more likely to end up on intensive care if you get Covid-19 than if you are white.

Why? Although people from a BAME background are more likely to live in poor, crowded housing and have worse health (higher rates of hypertension and type 2 diabetes), that does not explain why Covid-19 impacts this group so much worse than the flu does.

A study by the UK Office of National Statistics, which looked at the ethnic background of those who died from Covid-19, came to similar puzzling conclusions.[8]

They found that men and women from a black ethnic background are four times more likely to die from Covid-19 than those who are white. And that, even when you take into account things like social disadvantage and underlying disease, those of black ethnicity are still at nearly twice the risk.

The study also found that people from a Bangladeshi or Pakistani ethnic group were 1.7 times more likely to have a Covid-19-related death than whites.

They concluded that "the difference between ethnic groups in Covid-19 mortality is partly a result of socio-economic disadvantage and other circumstances, but a remaining part of the difference has not yet been explained."

It is an area where we really don't have proper answers at the moment, and should be a research priority.

2 How the virus escaped

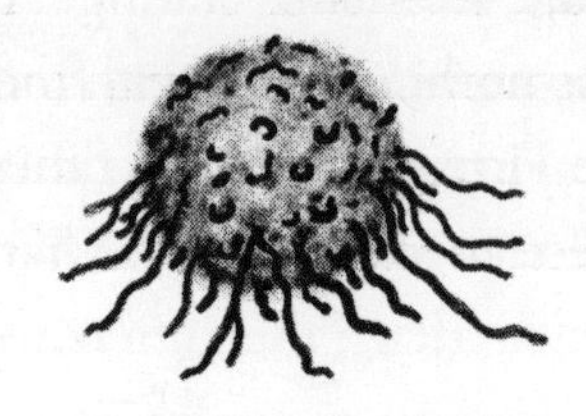

We don't know for sure where or when SARS-CoV-2 first jumped into a human. The official line is that it happened in a food market in Wuhan, China, in late 2019. This sounds plausible but one problem with this version of events is that a study of the earliest Covid-19 patients shows that many of them have no connection with the market.[9]

Another theory, which is fiercely disputed by the Chinese, is that the virus escaped from the Wuhan Institute of Virology, a high-security biolab where scientists had been studying novel coronaviruses.[10] In 2018, American scientists who visited the lab were so concerned that they sent warnings back to the US saying the lab's work on coronaviruses could cause a new SARS-like pandemic.

The head of the lab's bat-coronavirus research, Dr Shi Zhengli, denies her work had anything to do with the outbreak. She told reporters that the genomes of viruses from infected patients didn't match the viruses her team were working with. She is reported to have sent a WeChat message to friends stating, "I swear with my life, the virus has nothing to do with the lab."

However the virus first got out, this is what I have been able to piece together of what happened over the next 100 days.

Day 1

The first official notice that something was wrong came on December 31st, 2019, when the Chinese authorities in Wuhan, a city of 11 million people, told the World Health Organisation (WHO) that they had begun treating a number of patients with "pneumonia of unknown cause".

Day 2

In Wuhan many people celebrated January 1st, 2020, by visiting friends and relatives. An analysis of travel movements, based on mobile phone data, shows that on January 1st at least 175,000 people left Wuhan to travel to other parts of China. Hundreds more got on a plane and flew abroad.

Taiwan was one of the first countries to respond to the Chinese announcement that they had patients with a "pneumonia of unknown cause". The Taiwanese had suffered from the outbreak of SARS in 2002 and they feared a repeat. They contacted the WHO, asking for more information and on January 1st they began screening all passengers arriving from Wuhan with flu-like symptoms.

In Wuhan, fears about a deadly virus had by then already begun to circulate. The authorities reacted by cracking down on anyone they suspected of spreading "rumours", including a young ophthalmologist called Li Wenliang. His crime was that he had warned colleagues on WeChat about the presence in Wuhan of a SARS-like virus. Being an ophthalmologist (an expert in eyes) he was particularly concerned about the dangers of being up close and personal with infected patients and he suggested his colleagues take extra precautions to protect themselves from infection.

On January 3rd he was summoned to the Public Security Bureau where he was ordered to sign a letter confessing to making "false comments" that had "severely disturbed the social order".[11]

Day 10

On January 9th the Chinese announced that a 61-year

old man had died in a Wuhan after being infected by a novel coronavirus. But people were still allowed to travel freely.

According to one study, nearly 60,000 people, more than 800 of whom were infected with Covid-19, flew from Wuhan to cities outside China over the next two weeks.[12]

As well as flying to the US, UK, Europe and Australia, many travelled to cities in Asia, including Bangkok, where the first known overseas case of Covid-19 was caught by vigilant officials at Bangkok airport. She was a 61-year-old woman from Wuhan who had flown to Thailand on January 8th as part of a tour group. When she got on the plane she'd been struggling with a temperature and sore throat for four days, but she decided to travel anyway because she didn't want to miss out on her holiday.

When she and her group arrived at Bangkok airport they were screened by thermal cameras. Her raised temperature was picked up and she was immediately hospitalised. A test done a few days later confirmed that she was infected with the novel Wuhan virus.

Day 12

On January 11th the Chinese announced that they had managed to decode the full genetic blueprint of the novel coronavirus. This breakthrough was immediately shared with the rest of the world. It was an extraordinary scientific achievement that would inspire would-be vaccine makers everywhere, including Professor Robin Shattock, from Imperial College, London (see chapter 5), to spring into action.

But the Chinese government were still saying that there was no clear evidence of human-to-human transmission. This claim was publicly echoed by the WHO, who issued a statement on January 12th.[13] In it they said, "At this stage, there is no infection among healthcare workers, and no clear evidence of human to human transmission". They went on to add that countries should not start putting in place "any travel or trade restrictions on China".

Day 15

The head of China's National Health Commission, Ma Xiaowei, warned provincial health officials that this outbreak was likely to be major, at least on a par with SARS.[14] But it would be another six days before the public were officially warned about this threat.

During those six days tens of millions of Chinese took to the roads and skies to begin celebrating Chinese New Year.

Day 21

On January 20th President Xi said on television that there was an outbreak and it "must be taken seriously". By now it was becoming increasingly obvious just how infectious the virus really was.

Chinese scientists published a paper suggesting that the virus had an infectivity rate, R0, of around 2.5, meaning that anyone infected by it was likely to infect 2.5 others. Which doesn't sound that scary, until you do the maths. If you assume that it takes roughly five days for someone to go from being infected to infecting 2.5 others, you find that within a month a single infected person can have led to over 400 other people getting infected.

It was also becoming clear that some people could become infected without having any symptoms. Researchers from the University of Hong Kong published a study of a Chinese family who had been on holiday to Wuhan and became sick afterwards. All six members of the family had tested positive for the virus and CAT scans showed it had spread to their lungs, with evidence of "ground-glass changes" (see page 36). But, though five of the family reported having a fever, dry cough and diarrhoea, one of them, a ten-year-old child, had no symptoms at all. Despite being infected he remained perfectly healthy throughout.[15]

Alarmed by these new findings, the Chinese authorities put Wuhan into lockdown. They closed the airport and shut down bus and train services. They shut off a city of 11 million people. It was an extraordinary public health experiment; something like this had never been attempted before. But it was too late. The virus had already escaped.

Day 26

On January 25th Australia reported its first case of someone with Covid-19 infection. It was a man in his 50s from Wuhan, who had flown into Melbourne on January 19th, just a few days before Australia introduced heightened screening at the airport. A few days after arriving he felt ill, went to hospital and was immediately isolated.

Day 31

On January 30th the WHO declared that this outbreak was now a "public health emergency of international concern". The director general of the WHO, Dr Tedros Adhanom Ghebreyesus, said, "So far we have not seen any deaths outside China, for which we must be grateful. Although these numbers are relatively small compared to the number of cases in China, we must act together now to limit further spread."

Day 32

The following day, January 31st, the US announced it was closing its borders to any non-Americans who had recently been in China. As far as President Trump was concerned, that was job done. In an interview a few days later he said, "We pretty much shut it down coming in from China."

The trouble was, his travel ban turned out to be extremely leaky. According to *The New York Times* at least 430,000 people travelled on direct flights from China to the US in the first three months of 2020, "including nearly 40,000 in the two months after President Trump imposed restrictions on such travel".[16]

It seemed, anyway, to be a case of slamming the stable door closed after the horse has bolted. By the time Trump imposed a travel ban on travellers from China, the virus was already established in the US. One of the earliest known victims was a 57-year-old woman from Silicon Valley who developed flu-like symptoms and abruptly died on February 6th. Post-mortem tests showed she had Covid-19, despite having no known connections with China.

And China was no longer the only threat. People infected by Covid-19 had started to arrive in increasing numbers on the East coast of America, mainly travellers from Europe. They would spread the virus, unsuspected, through New York. There would be no ban on European travellers for another six weeks.

Day 39

On February 7th Li Wenliang, the young opthamologist who in December had tried to warn others of the threat from this new corononavirus, died after being infected by a patient. He was 34 years old and married with a young son. At the time of his death, his wife was pregnant with their second child. He was hailed as a hero and mourned right across China. Tragic though his death was, he was just one of hundreds of doctors, nurses, paramedics and other carers who would perish over the next few months.

Day 43

February 11th. The new viral infection was given a name: Covid-19, short for "coronavirus disease 2019".

Day 48

I'd been following the unfolding story of this epidemic with increasing alarm and on February 16th I wrote a column for a national newspaper, *The Mail on Sunday*, entitled "How to beat coronavirus? Sing Happy Birthday as you wash your hands".

It was obvious to me that this coronavirus was no longer a distant threat and it was time to start taking precautions. I suggested in my column that people should avoid shaking hands, hugging others and that we should all wash our hands as often as possible for as long as it takes to sing "Happy Birthday to You" twice.

Others were clearly less concerned. President Donald Trump told his fellow Americans, "We have it totally under control. It's going to be just fine." He optimistically added, "There's a theory that, in April, when it gets warm – historically, that has been able to kill the virus."

Day 51

Despite the looming threat, major sporting events in Europe were allowed to continue. On February 19th thousands of Spanish fans mixed with 40,000 Italian supporters for a Champions League game in Bergamo, Italy. The mayor, Giorgio Gori, later described that match as "the biological bomb" which exploded the virus all over the north of Italy. Spanish fans, who travelled to watch the game, took the virus home with them.

In the UK, scientists from Imperial College were asked to model a "Reasonable Worst Case". The questions the government wanted answered included, "If it takes off in the UK, what proportion of the population will be infected?" and "How many will need hospital care and a ventilator?"

It was a big ask, because at the time there were just nine cases of Covid-19 in the UK with no deaths. The best guess was that around 80% of people who got infected would have few, if any symptoms, but 5% might need to go into hospital and need intensive care.

Day 57

On February 25th the number of confirmed cases outside China outnumbered those inside China for the first time. The virus was spreading rapidly around the globe.

In the US, tens of thousands of people crammed the streets of New Orleans in an exuberant celebration of Mardi Gras. These celebrations helped spread the coronavirus like wildfire. Two months later New Orleans would have one of the highest per capita death rates in America.

As deaths mounted in Italy, it became the first place in Europe to introduce a "lockdown". The Italian government created "red zones" around towns in the north, quarantining more than 50,000 people. Schools were closed, sporting events cancelled. The mayor of Milan, however, decided to keep bars and restaurants open and to encourage tourists to visit the city's cathedral and museums.

In a similar spirit of misguided optimism, President Donald Trump tweeted, "The coronavirus is very much under control in the USA. Stock market starting to look very good to me!"

Within days, stock markets around the world fell.

Day 60

On February 28th Sub-Saharan Africa had its first confirmed case when an Italian citizen, who had returned to Nigeria from Milan, tested positive for the virus.

Day 64

By March 3rd hundreds of Italians had died from Covid-19 and Italian hospitals were beginning to buckle under the pressure of so many sick and elderly patients.

In the UK the British Prime Minister, Boris Johnson, had clearly not yet fully bought into the idea of social distancing. He said, at a press conference, "I was at a hospital the other night where I think there were a few coronavirus patients and I shook hands with everybody."

Day 72

On March 11th the WHO acknowledged that the virus

was spreading uncontrollably and that the world was in the grip of a serious pandemic.

Despite this, the organisers of the Cheltenham festival decided it was a good idea to allow 250,000 people from all over the UK and Ireland to cram together at the races for four days, many of them packed cheek by jowl in the crowded terraces and bars. Hospitals in the local area later recorded twice the number of deaths as those in other parts of the south west.

Day 77

On March 16th researchers from Imperial College, London, published an influential study which suggested that a "do-nothing" policy meant at least 510,000 people in the UK would die, along with 2.2 million Americans.[17]

They recommended a policy of "suppression," to slow down the spread of the virus and allow the struggling NHS to cope. "Flattening the curve" would mean closing schools, universities and businesses, and confining people to their homes.

Day 84

A week later, on March 23rd, Boris Johnson put the UK into lockdown. All non-essential businesses were to close and people were told that they would only be allowed to leave their homes for limited reasons, such as shopping for food, going out for exercise once a day, and travelling for work "if absolutely necessary".

By then most other European countries had gone into lockdown.

12th March	Norway and Ireland
13th March	Denmark and Poland
14th March	Spain
17th March	France
18th March	Belgium
20th March	Germany
23rd March	Greece and the UK

In the US, California and New York State had already declared a state of lockdown. Other states would soon follow.

New Zealand closed its borders to all non-residents on March 19th and Australia did the same on March 20th.

Ironically enough, just as the epidemic was taking off in the rest of the world, it began to lose momentum in China. On March 23rd the Chinese authorities announced that, for the first time, there had been no new cases of Covid-19.

Day 86

On March 25th the countdown clock to the 2020 Olympics was stopped and the organisers accepted that there could be no Olympic Games in July. The Games had only been cancelled three times, each time because of war. India, the world's largest democracy, put its 1.3 billion people into lockdown.

Day 87

On March 26th experts from Imperial College published an updated study which suggested that, with social distancing and measures to protect the vulnerable, global deaths from the virus could be cut from 40 million to less than 10 million.[18]

Day 94

On April 2nd the number of confirmed cases of Covid-19 passed the million mark. At least 50,000 people had died. Within two weeks both those numbers would double.

Day 100

After coming down with Covid-19, Boris Johnson was moved to intensive care. There was real concern as to whether he would survive. Although reasonably fit, he is in his 50s, male and overweight, all of which are risk factors.

America was now the epicentre of the pandemic and more than 2000 people were dying every day. Millions were forced to apply for unemployment benefits. Economists working for the bank JP Morgan predicted the American economy would shrink by 40% over the next few months and more than 20 million people would lose their jobs

On day 100, the Chinese announced that they had begun to bring people out of lockdown. Wuhan, where it all began, was now open for business.

3 Questions and Answers

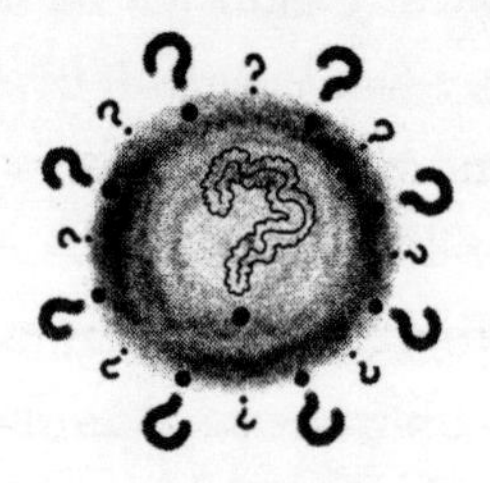

I have been asked lots of questions, mainly via my twitter account (@DrMichaelMosley), but also by friends and relatives who knew I was writing this book. Here are some of them.

How common are viruses?

Viruses are found almost everywhere on Earth, from the deepest oceans to the driest deserts. Wherever there are living creatures, they are present. Despite being so tiny (they are a million times smaller than a human cell) together they weigh more than every living thing on earth, including all plants, insects and animals. In fact someone with time on their hands calculated that if you were to string together just those viruses that live in the oceans they would reach to the planet Mars, and back again, more than 12 trillion times.[19]

The sea is full of them. According to Jennifer Brum, an oceanographer at Louisiana State University in Baton Rouge, there are around 200 million viruses in every mouthful of seawater you swallow when swimming in the ocean.

The reason we don't get sick more often is that, though there are millions of different species of virus out there, only a few hundred make us seriously ill.

The extraordinary thing about viruses is not only can they hijack our bodies to do their dirty work, but over time they have inserted themselves into our genome (the human blueprint that makes us who we are and which we hand down to our children). It's estimated that around 8% of the human genome is made up of viral DNA, which means that our cells are hard at work producing proteins for our viral "guests", for purposes that, for now, we can only guess at.

Are there "good" viruses?

Just as we've discovered in recent years how important certain "good" bacteria in our guts (the gut microbiome) are for our mental and physical health, so we are discovering that some of the viruses we are infected with are essential for our very existence. There are vital parts of our immune system, for example, which we use to fight off viruses, that originally came from other viruses.[20]

How often does a dangerous new virus, like Covid-19, emerge and cause a pandemic?

Novel viruses are infecting humans all the time, but most don't go anywhere. That is why a serious outbreak, caused by a novel virus, is not that common, though in recent years they have become more common. I've already mentioned SARS and MERS, but the most disturbing outbreak in my professional lifetime (before Covid-19) was the emergence of HIV (Human Immunodeficiency Virus), the virus that causes AIDS.

I saw a case of AIDS in 1984, when I was a medical student, and I was deeply shocked by how quickly and brutally it killed a previously healthy young man. Since it was first identified in 1983, HIV has killed more than 32 million people worldwide. And it hasn't gone away.

These days AIDS rarely makes the news, but 1.7 million people still get infected with it every year, mainly young people and children. A friend of mine, who is a dermatologist in Australia, says she is seeing increasing numbers, as people become complacent about the risks.

The good news is that because HIV is spread mainly through blood and semen, it is nothing like as infectious as an airborne virus. The bad news is that despite more than 30 years of trying, there is no vaccine, though drugs can be very effective.

One thing we know for certain is that new, dangerous viruses will continue to emerge. We can only hope that next time the world will be better prepared.

How many human coronaviruses are there?

The first human coronanavirus was identified by a Scottish researcher called June Almeida. In 1960 she was sent nasal washings from a child at a boarding school in Surrey who had had a cold. She looked at the sample down her electron microscope and saw viruses which looked a bit like the influenza virus, but which appeared to have a crown or halo. She and her colleagues at St Thomas's hospital in London called it a "coronavirus" because of the crown.

Since then scientists have identified four types of coronaviruses that can cause a mild cold, and three types that are deadly – those that cause SARS and MERS, and now Covid-19.

How is this new virus different from the coronaviruses that cause SARS or MERS?

One of the key differences is that when you get infected with Covid-19 you can soon be shedding lots of viruses without knowing you are infected. Viral shedding seems to occur early on in an infection (typically two to three days after getting infected), and most people (roughly 80%) get such mild symptoms that they ignore it. At least 40% of people who get Covid-19 have no symptoms at all. That is what allowed Covid-19 to spread so far and so fast. Early on in the pandemic there were a lot of people getting on planes and going out to work blissfully unaware that they were infected. Most governments were far too slow to react.

The other thing that seems to be different about this virus is that it is much more infectious than MERS or SARS. That is partly because it normally starts by infecting your upper throat, so that when you cough or sneeze you expel a lot of viruses into your surroundings, where they can be picked up by others. The other thing is that this virus seems to bind much more tightly to human cells than the viruses that cause SARS or MERS, so you need to inhale less of them to get infected.

It could have been worse. If you allow it to spread unhindered, then each person with Covid-19 infects on average 2.5 other people. For a disease like measles, which is transmitted largely by sneezing, the equivalent number is 18! If we didn't have a vaccine for measles any new outbreak would spread even more rapidly and kill even more people. The tragedy is that despite the fact that we have a really effective vaccine, measles is still killing thousands of children every year, in part because of the lies spread by deranged anti-vaxxers. I can only hope that, confronted by a virus to which we currently have no vaccine, people will come to appreciate what a wonderful gift vaccination is.

Was this virus made in a lab?

There is no evidence that Covid-19 is man-made. The likeliest explanation is it jumped from a bat, into a pangolin and then to a human. It is possible, though this is far more contentious, that it was being studied in a lab in China and then escaped.

How does Covid-19 spread?

The main way it spreads is through coughs or sneezes. If you have Covid-19 and cough while on a train or in a shop, small droplets containing millions of viruses will spray out of your nose or mouth. Some will hang around in the air, most will fall to the ground or nearby surfaces. If you cough into your hand, and then open a door or push a shopping trolley, then millions of viruses will transfer to that surface. If someone else comes along and uses that shopping trolley before it can be wiped down, then it will transfer to their hands. If they touch their nose or rub their eyes before washing their hands they may well get infected.

Studies suggest that, indoors, the Covid-19 virus can live for many hours on plastic or hard surfaces. So you could pick it up off a door handle, an ATM machine or a self-checkout terminal at a supermarket. It is a good idea, whenever you have been out, to wash your hands on coming home.

Where are the most likely places to get infected?

The place you are most likely to get infected is in your home, from a friend or member of your family who has brought it into your household. That's because when you are home you are indoors, with lots of face-to-face contact.

After that, the most likely place to get infected is in an enclosed space, with other people around, like a bar, restaurant, on public transport or in an office. Churches, as we've seen on page 27, are also potential Covid-19 death traps.

Thanks to smart detective work Chinese researchers have been able to show just how easily the virus can spread in a restaurant.[21] The drawing below represents the layout of a single room in a restaurant in Guangzhou, China. On January 24th the person who I have labelled A1, and who at the time did not have any symptoms, flew into Guangzhou from Wuhan and had lunch with his family.

Later that evening he felt ill and went to the local hospital, where he tested positive for Covid 19. Within a week four other members of his family had also tested positive for Covid-19, as did five other people who had been in the restaurant at the same time and who had been seated at tables B and C.

The restaurant was well ventilated, with an air-conditioner and an extractor fan. No one seated at tables E or F seems to have become infected, perhaps because they were out of the main airflow.

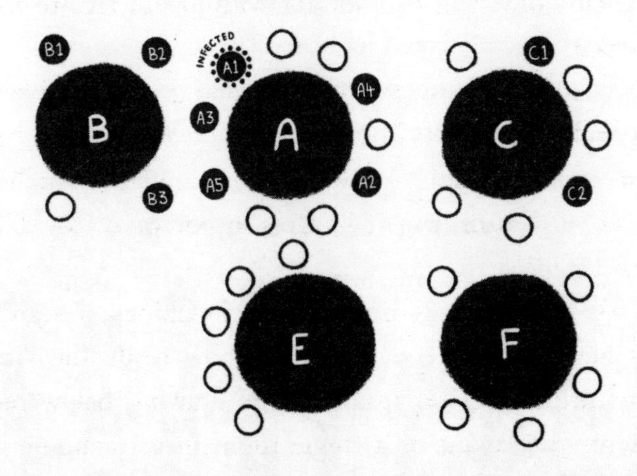

In another fascinating study, this time at a busy call centre, South Korean researchers showed how a single, asymptomatic employee, was able to infect nearly 100 others.[22] The investigation started when somone working in a 19-story office building went down with Covid-19. The Korea Centers for Disease Control and Prevention (KCDC) sprang into action. They closed the building down and sent in a team to test everyone who worked in the building, or who had visited.

Out of the 1,143 people they tracked and tested, 97 were positive for the virus. Of these, 94 had been working on the 11th floor of the building. In fact it turned out that nearly half the people working on that floor had got infected, almost all of whom were working in a single room (see below; the shaded seats represent where those who got infected had been sitting).

Thanks to prompt testing and isolation this particular outbreak was almost immediately snuffed out.

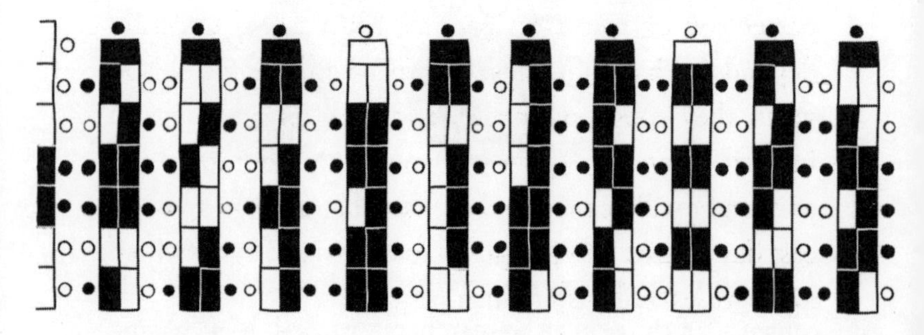

What about checking people's temperature before they're allowed on public transport or into a restaurant?

The problem with relying on temperature is that a lot of people who are infected don't have any symptoms. And even if you do have symptoms they won't necessarily include having a fever. So temperature checking will miss around half the people who actually have active Covid-19.

The other thing is, if you really want to accurately measure someone's temperature, you need to use a thermometer. Scanners measure skin temperature which can be quite different from your core temperature. If you have hot flushes or have just come from a brisk walk in the sun you will probably fail the scanner test.

Can I get it walking down the street?

You are very unlikely to get it from someone else who passes you on the street because your risk of infection depends both on how close you to are an infected person when they cough or sneeze, and how long you spend in their company. When you are walking outdoors any encounter will be brief and the fact that even on an overcast day you are being exposed to ultraviolet light (which kills viruses) will also reduce your risk.

Will warmer weather slow the spread of Covid 19?

Viruses generally prefer the cold, which is why you get a temperature when you have an infection. Raising your core temperature is your body's way of trying to stop the virus spreading.

As I mentioned above, there is good evidence that the Covid-19 virus does not survive long when exposed to UV light. Experiments carried out by the National Biodefense Analysis and Countermeasures Center have shown that direct sunlight swiftly destroys it.[23]

In a White House briefing, Bill Bryan, the acting Homeland Security undersecretary for science and technology, said, "Our most striking observation to date is the powerful effect that solar light appears to have on killing the virus – both surfaces and in the air. We've seen a similar effect with both temperature and humidity as well, where increasing the temperature and humidity or both is generally less favorable to the virus."

The reason why bright sunlight kills viruses is because the ultraviolet component in sunlight can destroy the sort of fragile DNA or RNA that viruses contain. It doesn't mean you can't pick up an infection outdoors on a sunny day, but it is far less likely than inside a shop, restaurant or office.

If Covid-19 behaves anything like the flu, it will get much worse in winter.

Can pets, like cats and dogs, get and spread the new coronavirus?

There have been a number of confirmed cases of cats coming down with Covid-19, as well as lions and tigers at a New York zoo. When cats become infected they get mild respiratory symptoms and then recover. There is no evidence that pets can give Covid-19 to their owners. In one family, the cat got Covid-19 but none of the family did (which begs the question of where the cat got it from).

Should I wear a mask when I am outside?

This is a big one. Wearing proper masks if you are in a hospital setting is obviously essential, but what about when you are on your way to the shops? One of the clear differences between countries that controlled the initial spread of the virus, like China, South Korea and Taiwan, and countries that didn't was the fact that in the former countries people were actively encouraged to wear masks outdoors. One study suggested that if just 60% of people could be persuaded to wear masks then that alone could stop the pandemic.

The masks don't have to be that sophisticated. Professor Trish Greenhalgh and research scientist Jeremy Howard recently carried out a comprehensive review on face masks and concluded that a basic mask made out of an old T-shirt combined with kitchen paper would be good enough.[24]

The reason why wearing simple homemade masks has such a big impact on transmission of the virus is not so much because they will protect the wearer (though they might, particularly if someone coughs directly in your face), but more because they will dramatically reduce the amount of droplets someone who is infected will spray around if they happen to have Covid-19.

The superpower that this virus possesses is its ability to infect your throat and make you into a superspreader long before you realise you are infected. What wearing a mask out in public does is dramatically reduce that risk.

In fact, as Trish Greenhalgh and Jeremy Howard point out, "If you have Covid-19 and cough on someone from eight inches away, wearing a cotton mask will reduce the amount of virus you transmit to that person by 36 times."

So if you wear a mask there is a chance that you will be saving a lot of lives. Unfortunately, most people are not that altruistic. Since it is unlikely that that enough people can be persuaded, voluntarily, to wear a mask, it is likely that most governments will have to go down the route of making wearing them compulsory. This is what happened in the Spanish flu outbreak of 1918 which killed at least 50 million people. In the US the police came down so hard on people seen outdoors without a mask that this in itself led to several deaths, with people being shot dead on the street.

If you are making your own mask it is a good idea to use a tightly woven fabric that you can still breathe through. To make your own simple mask and for everything you could want to find out about mask making and mask cleaning, I recommend visiting https://masks4all.co/how-to-make-a-homemade-mask/

What is the best protection against the virus?

The best way of protecting yourself is by washing your hands, often and thoroughly, with soap, particularly after you have been out in public.

What about taking vitamin C supplements ?

There is absolutely no evidence that taking vitamin C supplements will help protect you against Covid-19. Nor will Echinacea, drinking green tea or zinc supplements. Nor raw garlic.

I am a fan of garlic, as part of the Mediterranean diet, but the only way that eating raw garlic is likely to help is by discouraging others from coming too close to you.

And there are dangers to overdoing it. I read a story in the newspaper about a woman who had to go into hospital with a severely inflamed throat after eating 1.5kg of raw garlic.

What should I do if I think I might have Covid-19?

If you have mild symptoms then you should self-isolate and treat it like the flu. Get plenty of sleep, drink plenty of fluid and, if you have a temperature, take paracetamol. 80% of people, after a mild illness, get better. Another 15% get quite ill with shortness of breath, joint pain and fevers, but recover over the course of a couple of weeks. Less than 5% need to go into hospital.

What if somebody in my family gets sick?

When my son Dan came down with Covid-19 we asked him to stay in his room and wear a mask if he absolutely had to come out. We left his food on a tray outside his room and we were careful to wash his dishes separately, using gloves. We also cleaned all the surfaces he might have touched. We were lucky we didn't have to share a bathroom and he kept himself amused with his mobile phone and laptop. Fortunately, he recovered fast and none of us came down with anything, though it did mean we had to self-isolate for a couple of weeks. He lost his sense of smell and taste, which happens to many people with Covid-19, but they both slowly came back over the next few weeks.

What if I have more serious symptoms?

People who become seriously ill often have a continuous cough and then, about a week into the infection, they suddenly find it hard to breathe and become really quite ill. This is mainly because the body's immune system has started to kick in, and has overreacted. What you are experiencing is the collateral damage caused by your immune system taking on the virus. If you start getting severe shortness of breath, difficulty breathing or blue lips, this is a sign that your oxygen saturation levels are falling dangerously low and you need to be seen urgently.

What happens if I need intensive care?

Once you are in hospital the staff will decide whether to put you on oxygen, or put you on a ventilator. The latter means you will need to be intubated and your chances of survival are not much better than 50;50. Even if you survive it may take over a year to recover and you will almost certainly require physiotherapy. You may also need psychological support because of the high incidence of post traumatic stress disorder (PTSD).

What drug treatments are available?

At the time of writing we don't have any drug treatments that are really effective. One of the more promising is remdesivir, an antiviral drug that was first developed years ago to fight Ebola. It didn't work that well against Ebola, but tests done in the lab suggest it may help prevent the Covid-19 virus from replicating. There has been one randomised controlled trial which showed that, on average, it reduces the time it takes to recover from Covid 19 from 15 days to 11 days. There was also a modest impact on the risk of dying, though this was not statistically significant.[25]

Another drug, which got a lot of attention from US President Donald Trump after a small study done in France suggested it might be of benefit, is the anti-malaria drug hydroxychloroquine. Unfortunately, it has significant side effects and a study which looked at its impact on 368 American military veterans hospitalised with Covid-19 found that more than twice as many died after being given the drug than those who got usual care.[26]

Another way to fight the virus is by using human antibodies, collected from the blood of people who have had the virus and survived. This approach has been used to save lives during polio and Ebola epidemics, but we don't know yet how well it will work with Covid-19. Since one survivor can only donate enough blood to help two sick people it is clearly rather limited in its use, so companies are now looking at ways to produce artificial antibodies.

To try and get answers, fast, the WHO has set up a huge international trial – the Solidarity Trial – which is testing four different drug regimes in over 100 different countries. When a patient comes in they are randomly allocated to one of the trial drugs or to standard hospital care. The four drug regimes being tested are remdesivir and hydroxychloroquine, mentioned above, plus:

- Lopinavir and ritonavir, antiviral drugs which have been successfully used against AIDS
- Lopinavir/ritonavir combined with interferon-beta, a drug that helps reduce inflammation.

With the global death toll mounting, the world is desperate for effective treatments. But at the moment there is no obvious cure on the horizon.

If I have had Covid-19 can I catch it again?

It is too early to say but in the short term it seems unlikely that someone who has had the virus and recovered will come down with Covid-19 again. The reason why people can get the flu more than once is because flu viruses are constantly mutating and changing in a way that this virus doesn't seem to be doing. Stories of people being infected, recovering and then getting infected again are more likely due to faulty testing than a faulty immune response.

What sort of tests are there?

There is the RT-PCR test. This looks for the presence of the virus – ie whether you are currently infected with it, symptoms or not. The test works by detecting tiny fragments of viral genetic material. Normally it will involve swabbing the inside of your nose and the back of your throat. Unless it is done properly you get a lot of false negatives – ie people are told they don't have it when they do. That is because you have missed the actual areas that are infected.

You can also get false positives, where you are told you are still infected when you are not. That is because it detects viral fragments and can't tell you if those viruses are still active. Even when your viral infection is over, you can still have fragments of dead viral genetic material floating around.

The other test looks for antibodies to the Covid-19 virus. Your body normally starts to produce antibodies to a novel virus within ten days and levels should remain raised for at least several months.

Which countries have handled this crisis really well?

South Korea, Taiwan, China, New Zealand and Australia have all been very effective at squashing the curve and getting rates of infection under control without too many deaths. South Korea and Taiwan did it by doing lots of testing, aggressively tracing contacts of people who are infected, and then making sure they self-isolate. From early on they were checking the body temperatures of all incoming and outgoing passengers at train stations and other places. Officials operated drive-through testing centres and sent out mobile phone alerts to citizens when new cases were reported in their districts.

Australia and New Zealand got on top of the virus by closing their borders, imposing social distancing and doing widespread testing.

China imposed strict travel limitations and they required people to wear masks at all times outdoors. They also imposed a regime of temperature checking at the doors of office buildings, stores, restaurants, hotels, apartments and public transit stations.

Will the virus come back once the number of new cases drops off?

It is likely that most countries will see new outbreaks

once social distancing is lifted. The 1918 pandemic flu circled the world in three waves, with the second wave being an even bigger killer than the first. But until we see what actually happens, we don't know how Covid-19 will behave.

Might the new virus "burn out" like other viral outbreaks have done?

I would love to be able to say yes, but I think that it is unlikely. Covid-19 is already too well established around the world. The virus that caused SARS came and went, and the virus that caused MERS never really took off. Unless we get a vaccine, Covid-19, like the influenza virus that causes the seasonal flu, is likely be with us for a long, long time. It's possible that it could mutate into a less dangerous form so that fewer people die from it, as happened before with the swine flu in 2009. But I wouldn't count on it.

4 How to bolster your immune system

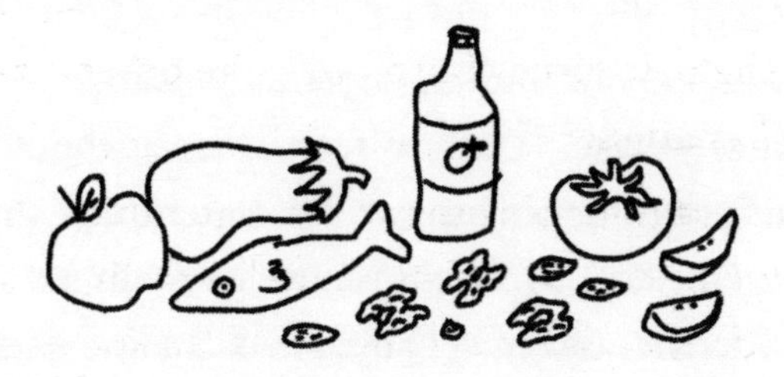

The best way to protect yourself and your family from being infected by the Covid-19 virus is by regular handwashing and social distancing. But keeping the virus at bay is going to be really hard in the months ahead, particularly when those of us who live in the Northern hemisphere go into winter. That is when we can expect a second wave of infections, which may be worse than what we have seen so far. The lesson from the 1918 outbreak of Spanish flu was that the first wave was bad, the second wave (which began around September) was horrendous.

I'm hoping for a vaccine as soon as possible, but being realistic it is unlikely that it will be widely available before 2021. Until then it is vitally important to do what you can to support your immune system so it is in good shape if and when it has to do battle with the virus.

Your immune system faces a tricky balancing act. It has to respond to threats, but not go too far. One of the reasons why older people are dying in such large numbers is because our immune system tends to become less efficient as we age. It fails to react when it should, then overreacts causing extensive collateral damage.

An ageing and inefficient immune system is not inevitable. There are lifestyle changes that can keep it in good shape, even when you get older.

So what has been shown to work? Broadly, the things you can do fall into seven categories, all of which overlap and reinforce each other.

1/. Shrink your waist

If you have a large waist then you are at much greater risk of becoming seriously ill if you get Covid-19. Why? It is partly because the more overweight you are, the lower your lung capacity. So if Covid-19 attacks your lungs you are more likely to end up in intensive care.

People with excess fat also tend to have a less efficient immune response. This means they not only get more infections but vaccines are less effective. A study of more than a thousand people given a flu jab found that the people who were obese were twice as likely to get the flu, despite being vaccinated, as those who were slimmer.[27]

Another reason why you might want to shrink your waist, ASAP, is because a large waist often goes hand in hand with raised blood sugar levels. People with type 2 diabetes or prediabetes (where your blood sugars are raised but not yet in the diabetic range) are more prone to getting infections. Amongst other things, raised blood sugar unleashes destructive molecules called dicarbonyls (the breakdown products of glucose) that interfere with the body's natural infection-control defences.

One of the best ways to lose gut fat, and bring your blood sugar levels down fast and safely, is with an 800-calorie rapid weight loss diet. There is good evidence from big, randomised trials, that an 800-calorie diet is also one of the best ways to reverse type 2 diabetes and rid yourself of metabolic syndrome (see page 88).

2/. Try intermittent fasting

Intermittent fasting, where you cut your calories a couple of days a week, is a popular way to lose weight. The 5:2 diet (which I'm famous for) and Time Restricted Eating, where you only eat within a 10-hour window each day, have both been shown to help people lose weight. But intermittent fasting has other health benefits, including potentially helping improve your immune system. More on that in a moment.

3/. Eat a more Mediterranean-style diet
The traditional diet of Mediterranean countries, rich in olive oil, nuts, oily fish and legumes, is regularly voted by health professionals as the healthiest diet on the planet. Changing the way you eat will not only reduce your risk of metabolic disease but should help support your immune system.

4/. Boost your microbiome
One of the reasons why the Mediterranean diet is so super healthy is because it boosts levels of the "good" microbes in your gut. This, in turn, has been shown to play an important role in the body's immune response to infectious pathogens.

5/. Improve your sleep
We know that getting good quality sleep is essential for the production and release of key components of your immune system and there is strong evidence that getting a good night's sleep is a great way to keep infections at bay. Some top sleep tips coming up.

6/. Become more active
Regular physical activity is good for your heart, your

bones and your muscles. It can also improve your mood. But what I find particularly encouraging right now is evidence that just 20 minutes a day is enough to give your immune system a good work out as well. The important thing, as I will reveal, is to get a decent mix of different exercises.

7/. Reduce stress

These are horribly stressful times and we know that chronic stress has a direct and damaging effect on your immune system. All the things I've just described, from losing weight to becoming more active and eating a Med-style diet, are great ways to reduce stress. But there are a few other tips I'm about to share which I personally have found really useful.

Shrink your waist

The Covid-19 virus seems almost selective about who it kills. Most people, particularly the young, shake it off while others become extremely ill. Significant risk factors include your age, having type 2 diabetes, high blood pressure, heart disease and being obese.

The usual measure of whether someone is overweight or obese is Body Mass Index. You calculate your BMI by taking your weight and dividing it by your height squared. I am 1.8 metres tall and weigh 80kg so my BMI = 80/(1.8x1.8) = 24.7

That puts me, just, in the healthy range. Having a BMI over 30 makes you "obese" and that doubles your risk of ending up in intensive care if you get Covid-19.

But BMI is a crude predictor of health. What is more important is not how much you weigh, but how much of that weight is fat and where it is stored. Fat on your bottom or hips seems to be relatively harmless. The most dangerous place to store fat (and you don't, of course, have any choice where it goes) is around your gut.

Fat in and around your gut is known as visceral fat. To measure it precisely you would need to have something called a DEXA scan, but a tape measure is almost as good. If your waist is much more than half your height then there is a good chance that you are carrying too much visceral fat.

Men are more likely to store fat around their gut than women, which may help explain why we are twice as likely to end up in intensive care if we get Covid-19.

Metabolic disease

The problem with visceral fat is that it is linked to a range of other chronic diseases, which come under the label metabolic syndrome. This is also known as syndrome X, insulin resistance syndrome or "The deadly quartet". That is because those with a large waist also commonly have raised blood sugar levels, hypertension and abnormal levels of cholesterol and fat in the blood.

Having metabolic syndrome is bad for you, at the best of times, but it is even more dangerous if you get Covid-19. That's because having chronic low-grade inflammation and insulin resistance (both characteristic of metabolic disease) impairs your immune response to pathogens. We know that obesity and diabetes, independently, make you vulnerable to Covid-19. Put them together, along with hypertension, and your risk levels shoot up.

According to a recent commentary in the respected science journal *Nature*, "patients with type 2 diabetes and metabolic syndrome might have to up 10 times greater risk of death when they contract Covid-19".

That figure is speculative, and may overstate the risk. But there's no doubt that there is a risk and that is worrying, particularly as more than 1 in 3 adults over the age of 50 in the UK, Australia and US have metabolic syndrome. Many of them don't know it.

If you want to shrink your waist, and get rid of metabolic disease, you can do it any way that suits you. But as I point out in my recent book, *The Fast 800*, your best bet may well be an 800-calorie rapid weight loss diet.

The Fast 800

Sticking to eating 800 calories a day, every day, for up to 12 weeks is a regimen that has been shown by several studies to be safe and to lead to substantial, sustained weight loss. In 2018 a study called DiRECT, run by Professor Roy Taylor from Newcastle University, showed that people with type 2 diabetes who were asked to go on an 800-calorie diet for a couple of months lost and kept off an average 10kg. Half were able to come off all diabetes medication.[28]

In 2018 researchers from Oxford University also published a study called DROPLET where 278 overweight or obese adults were either assigned to a regimen where they got 800 calories a day in the form of meal replacement shakes, or were put on a standard slow and steady diet programme.[29]

Those on the meal replacement regimen were asked to stick to it for eight weeks, before gradually switching to eating real food. At the end of a year the group on the rapid weight loss diet had lost and kept off an average of 10.7kg, while those in the standard dieting group had lost 3kg.

Susan Jebb, professor of diet and population health at Oxford University and the lead researcher, was delighted by the results. "It's phenomenal – extraordinary – like nothing we've seen in primary care before." She thinks one of the reasons that the rapid weight loss group did so well is because rapid weight loss is very motivating: "The excitement gets them through the first few difficult weeks... We need to capitalise on all that enthusiasm that people have at the beginning to really lose weight and get off as much weight as they possibly can."

Like other weight loss specialists I spoke to, she said that science did not support the often-repeated claims that people's metabolic rates will crash, never to recover, or that people who lose weight fast put it on even faster. Instead she said studies consistently show that early weight loss predicts long-term weight loss.

"Weight loss at four weeks, certainly at 12 weeks, is a really good predictor of what will happen later. In a previous study we showed that weight loss at 12 weeks predicted weight loss at two years."

Above all, Professor Jebb is frustrated by how slowly things are changing. "If we had a new drug which had achieved something similar it would be screamed from the roof tops… We have something which is effective and which is really cheap. And we are not doing it. I find that unbelievable."

More recently, another smaller study carried out by Oxford University, called Diamond, in which my wife, Dr Clare Bailey, was an author, showed that you could get similar impressive results from eating an 800-calorie, low-carb Med diet for a couple of months.[30]

If you want to find out more, and get ideas for suitable 800-calorie-a-day recipes, then do visit thefast800.com.

Is it safe to do a rapid weight loss programme, particularly now?

Losing weight, particularly if you need to shift a few inches from your waist, will cut your risk of metabolic disease and hopefully increase your chance of fighting off Covid-19. But are there risks to losing weight during this pandemic? I asked Professor Roy Taylor, who has been running rapid weight loss trials for some years now, what he thought.

"Studies to date", he told me, "have shown no negative impact on the immune system from rapid calorie restriction, as long as you are consuming adequate protein, vitamins, minerals and other micronutrients." He went on to add that the benefits would be seen quickly, particularly for those with raised blood sugar levels.

"If you decide to do rapid weight loss then this will result in rapid normalisation of your blood sugar levels and bring down your of risk of reacting badly to Covid-19 should you contract it, within days or weeks."

Try intermittent fasting

I appreciate that there are people who don't want to do a rapid weight loss approach, aren't suitable or don't want to do it for long. If you have tummy fat you want to lose I would still recommend a couple of weeks of rapid weight loss and then that you consider switching to what I call the 5:2 diet.

It is a form of intermittent fasting, where you cut your calories to 800 calories a day, but only for two days a week. It was a regime I came up with in 2012, when I discovered that I had type 2 diabetes. Using this approach I lost 9kg in less than eight weeks and returned my blood sugars to normal, without medication.

Since then a number of studies have shown it is an effective way to lose weight, and keep it off, but there is also evidence that this approach can improve the workings of your immune system.

In December 2019 there was a review paper published in the prestigious *New England Journal of Medicine* which looked at the benefits of two different approaches to intermittent fasting: the 5:2 or Time Restricted Eating, where you only eat within a restricted time window (such as from 10am to 8pm). They concluded that both approaches led to "improvements in blood pressure; resting heart rate; levels of HDL and LDL cholesterol, triglycerides, glucose, and insulin resistance. In addition, intermittent fasting reduces markers of systemic inflammation and oxidative stress that are associated with atherosclerosis."

"Systemic inflammation" means widespread inflammation throughout the body and it is a sign of a malfunctioning immune system. It means that your body is making too many pro-inflammatory cytokines and is a predictor of who will do badly when they get Covid-19.

Switch to a Mediterranean-style diet

Like any army, the soldiers of your immune system need to be properly fed if they are to be fighting fit. The recipes in all my books are based on a Mediterranean-style diet, a way of eating that is rich in healthy natural fats, nuts and fish, as well as veggies and legumes, which are packed with disease-fighting vitamins and minerals.

The reason I am such a fan of the Mediterranean diet is because it tastes great, but also because there is so much solid scientific evidence that adopting this lifestyle will cut your risk of heart disease, cancer, type 2 diabetes, depression and dementia. On top of that, thanks to recent studies, we know it can improve your sleep (see below) and improve the workings of your immune system, even if you are a bit older.[31]

One reason why this diet is so beneficial is because as well as nourishing us, it has a very positive effect on your gut microbiome – the trillions of microbes that live in your gut and which are so important for your physical and mental wellbeing. The Med diet is particularly effective at boosting levels of "good" bacteria in your gut, like Bifidobacterium and Lactobacillus. These turn the fibre and other nutrients in the Med diet into chemicals called short-chain fatty acids (SCFs), which reduce inflammation in the gut and throughout the body.

Reducing systemic inflammation, as I mentioned above, will not only reduce your risk of heart disease and cancer, but can mean you are less likely to experience a "cytokine storm", that dangerous overreaction by the immune system to Covid-19 that leads to serious damage to vital organs and sometimes to death.

To make your diet more "Mediterranean" and nourish your microbiome, it is important to start by cutting down on processed foods like snacks and ready meals, tempting though they may be during these stressful times. Eating lots of sugary or processed foods will just reinforce and feed the "bad" pro-inflammatory microbes that live in the gut.

Instead you should:

- Eat natural healthy fats in the form of real food, such as olive oil, salmon, tuna, full-fat dairy, avocado, nuts and seeds. These natural fats are also good for the waist and the heart, and will keep you feeling full for longer.
- Eat decent amounts of protein. This means eating generous amounts of foods such as oily fish, seafood, chicken, some red meat, eggs, tofu, beans, pulses, dairy and nuts. You need at least 50-60g of protein a day, every day. As you get older, you need more. That said, you should restrict your intake of processed meats such as sausages, bacon and salami, as these are not healthy sources of protein. Most contain high levels of salt, nitrates and other preservatives.
- Eat plenty of green and coloured veg. It is especially important to eat plenty of dark-green leafy vegetables, such as spinach, broccoli, cabbage, kale and salads, as well as coloured vegetables – these are very low in calories and contain many essential vitamins and nutrients. They also contain lots of fibre, which the "good" microbes in your gut will benefit from.
- Swap to wholegrains and pulses. Eat more "com-

plex carbohydrates", which are rich in fibre. This means swapping white pasta and rice for wholegrains and pulses such as lentils, beans, quinoa, wild rice and buckwheat. Choose multi-grain, seeded, sourdough or rye bread over white. Again, the good bacteria in your gut will thrive on the fibre in these foods.

- Avoid snacking between meals or late-night grazing. Grazing stops fat burning. If you must, snack on non-starchy vegetables such as broccoli, cucumber or celery, or a small handful of nuts or a small piece of cheese. Eating lots of fruit is not great, particularly when you are trying to lose weight.
- Drink healthily. Plenty of black tea, fruit or herbal tea, black coffee, water. As for alcohol, an occasional glass of red wine with a meal is okay but if you are doing an 800-calorie fast day, it's best to avoid alcohol altogether.
- As well as good quality food, the Mediterranean is famous for its sunshine, and there is mounting evidence that the sunshine vitamin, vitamin D, is important for making sure your immune system behaves optimally. So do make sure you get plenty of fresh air and if you have darker skin or spend a lot of time indoors then do take a vitamin D supplement.

The Mediterranean diet is more than just a diet. It's

about developing a set of habits and making permanent changes to your lifestyle. It involves cutting back on processed, ready-made and fast foods, and instead opting for whole-food meals cooked, where possible, from scratch. And it is about eating food slowly and enjoying it with family and friends. Too often we eat without taking the time to appreciate what is going in our mouths. So don't eat your meal in front of the TV. Make the effort to savour it fully.

Fermented foods

I am also a fan of fermented foods which are rich in probiotics, living bacteria. Although there is no direct evidence that they will benefit your immunity, they are a useful way of boosting your "good" bacteria. Some of my favourite fermented foods include sauerkraut, which is a form of fermented cabbage. My wife makes a really tasty sauerkraut using nothing but organic cabbage, salt and some beetroot for colour. You can also add turmeric or cumin. She also makes kimchi, a Korean dish of fermented cabbage with added chilli and ginger. You can find fermented food recipes at thefast800.com.

One note of caution: if you have not eaten fermented foods before, you should start with small amounts or you might get some gastrointestinal symptoms initially, like bloating or gas.

Sleep and the immune system

Anyone who has struggled with sleep will know what a big impact it has on memory, mood and concentration. What is less obvious is the impact that sleep has on your immune system. Yet numerous studies have also shown that there is a very clear link between poor sleep and vulnerability to viral infections.

One of the reasons why a good night's sleep is so important for the immune system is that it is while you are in deep sleep that your body makes cytokines, the proteins that start and co-ordinate your immune response to viral infections. Good-quality sleep is also important for the production of infection-fighting antibodies and T-killer cells.

The impact that sleep has on our ability to fight viral infections was highlighted by an extraordinary study done a few years ago, in which American researchers deliberately tried to infect a large group of healthy volunteers to see how well their immune systems responded.[32]

In this particular experiment researchers asked 164 healthy men and women to wear sleep trackers and keep a record of how well they slept. They were then brought into a lab and asked to inhale nasal droplets containing cold-inducing viruses.

The volunteers were then kept isolated from each other in a nearby hotel for another five days and constantly monitored. It turned out that those who slept less than six hours a night were four times more likely to get a cold than those who got seven hours or more.

So not getting enough sleep made them more vulnerable to the impact of the common cold virus, despite being exposed to the same level of infection.

If you suffer from poor sleep there are a number of tried and tested ways to improve your sleep quality which I describe in detail in my latest book, *Fast Asleep*. These include:

- Stick to a regular sleep window, ie follow a regular wake-up-go-to-bed routine. Try to stick to the same wake-up time every day of the week, including weekends.
- Manage your stressful thoughts by practising mindfulness and breathing exercises. I am a particular fan of a breathing exercise called 4:2:4. You breathe in through your nose to a count of four, hold your breath to a count of two, then breathe out to a count of four. Do this for a couple of minutes.
- Get out of bed if you can't sleep, and don't get back in until you feel tired. This is known as stimulus control, and the idea is that you have to learn to

associate "bed" with "sleep" and "sex" and nothing else.

- Expose yourself to bright light (daylight or by using a light box) first thing in the morning. This will help reset your circadian rhythms, your internal clock.
- Remain active and do plenty of resistance exercises, such as press-ups and squats.
- Eat a Mediterranean-style diet that includes fermented foods. There is plenty of evidence this will improve sleep quality by boosting levels of your "good" bacteria.
- If you have weight to lose, consider a rapid weight loss diet which will reduce snoring and can cure sleep apnoea (where your breathing stops and starts while you sleep), both of which can seriously disrupt your sleep.
- Try sleep restriction therapy. For more details on this visit fast-asleep.com.

Exercise and the immune system

In addition to eating healthily and getting a good night's sleep, it is important to go out in the fresh air and get active. I go for a 30-minute walk or run in nearby fields most mornings. It is partly to get my heart racing, but also so I can get in plenty of early-morning light and get my immune system into shape.

Researchers at University of California San Diego School of Medicine recently asked 47 volunteers to walk briskly on a treadmill at a moderate speed for 20 minutes. They collected blood before and after the volunteers exercised.

They found that 20 minutes was enough to reduce tumour necrosis factor (TNF), a cytokine that drives chronic inflammation. It was also enough to boost levels of an antioxidant known as "extracellular superoxide dismutase" (EcSOD). Both of these could help reduce the risk of acute respiratory distress syndrome (ARDS), a major cause of death in patients with Covid-19.[33]

As well as running, walking and some cycling, I also do strength exercises, such as press-ups and squats, most days. Although there is lots of evidence that regular exercise is good for the immune system, don't overdo it. There is always the risk that you will pull something (earlier this year I tore my Achilles tendon while running) and studies on mice suggest that a sudden increase in exercise intensity and volume can have a temporary negative effect on the immune system.

And finally, don't stress!

Being told "not to stress" is actually quite annoying. For most people stress is just a part of everyday life. In the short term it can help get you out of bed and get on with doing things that you don't want to do. But if it's chronic it will take a heavy toll on your immune system.

Chronic stress boosts levels of the hormone cortisol, which leads to chronic inflammation. It also reduces certain lymphocytes – the white blood cells that help fight off infection.

Fortunately, all the things I've recommended so far have been shown to reduce chronic stress:

- Losing weight will mean that you sleep better, which means you will be less likely to feel those sleep-deprived bingeing urges.
- Intermittent fasting, like the 5:2, has been shown to improve mood and reduce stress, possibly by boosting levels of a hormone called brain derived neurotrophic hormone (BDNF). This protects against the toxic effects of stress.
- Studies by the Food and Mood Centre in Australia have shown that going on a Med diet can have a big impact on levels of stress, anxiety and depression.
- Exercise is also a great stress-buster. It pumps up

the production of your brain's feel-good neuro-transmitters, including BDNF and endorphins.

On top of those I also recommend trying mindful meditation. Ten to 15 minutes a day, done three or four times a week, has been shown to reduce stress and cortisol levels.

There are more stress busting tips, as well as help with all the above, at thefast800.com.

5 The race for the vaccine

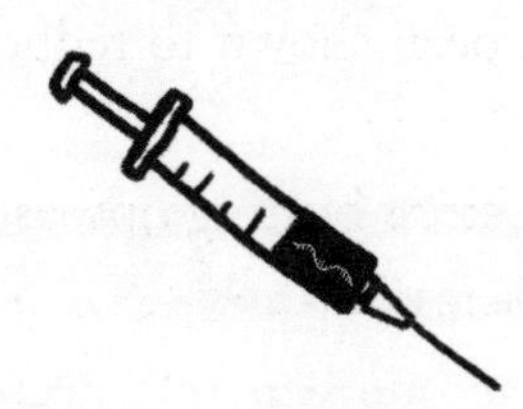

With a deadly new virus stalking the planet, the race to create a safe and effective vaccine is like nothing we've seen before. In record time more than a hundred vaccines have gone into development, several of which have already begun to be tested on humans. So what are the chances of success and what is the time scale?

The good news is that with so many vaccines against Covid-19 in play, and with so much money behind them, it is possible that at least one of them will come through the rigorous testing that is required if not by the end of 2020, certainly by 2021.

But there are huge challenges for the vaccine makers to overcome. Before describing some of the front runners, I would like to take a brief journey back into history and tell the story of how the first vaccine was used to contain and ultimately eradicate the greatest killer of all time. The lessons we've learnt from doing that will help us in our current battle.

Smallpox – the Speckled Monster

Three hundred years ago life expectancy in the developed world was less than half what it is today. People were killed in huge numbers by infectious diseases like typhoid, cholera and tuberculosis. In London more than 15% of babies died before their first birthday. The biggest killer was smallpox, the Speckled Monster.

Like Covid-19, smallpox could be spread by a cough or a sneeze. And, because the scabs and pus which oozed from a patient's sores contained lots of virus, you could also get smallpox by touching contaminated bedding or clothing.

When you first got smallpox you felt fine. After a week or so, you would start getting symptoms, such as fever, muscle aches, and nausea. Soon, starting in your mouth, tiny red spots would appear all over your body. These spots would turn to hard, pus-filled blisters which felt like gunshot pellets and which would then start to split away from the underlying skin, causing agonising pain. Sometimes the patient's skin would turn black and come off in strips.

If you got the most common form of smallpox, Variola major, then your chance of dying were around 30%. If you survived, there was a risk you would be left blind and hideously disfigured.

The origins

Smallpox jumped from animals into humans thousands of years ago, probably in Africa. Smallpox scars can be seen on the faces of 3000-year-old Egyptian mummies. From Africa the virus was carried by traders to the rest of the world.

Down the centuries it killed, blinded and scarred hundreds of millions of people. An outbreak in Japan in the 8th century killed one in three of the population. In the 20th century alone it was responsible for the deaths of at least 300 million people.

Smallpox killed rich and poor, emperors and kings, pharaohs and prophets. When Europeans first travelled to the Americas, they brought smallpox with them, wiping out an estimated 90% of the Aztecs and Incas. There was a similar tragic outcome when Europeans went to North America and Australia.

The smallpox virus still exists, but the only known samples are stored in liquid nitrogen and held in two high security facilities. One is in Russia, and the other in the Centres for Disease Control and Prevention in Atlanta. A few years ago I went there while making a film about smallpox.

The virus is still considered so dangerous that I was not allowed into the Level 4 bio-containment lab where they keep it. In fact I was told that only ten people in the world have clearance to handle it and to do so they first need to put on fully pressurised suits before passing through multiple computer-controlled airlocks.

Many people would like these surviving samples to be destroyed, to eliminate any possibility that the virus could escape; others argue that there is still much to learn from a scrap of genetic material that has killed more people than every other infectious disease, put together.

Smallpox is the only viral infection we have managed to eradicate. So how did we do it?

The Gloucester doctor

The hero of the smallpox vaccine story is an 18th-century English doctor called Edward Jenner. As a busy doctor he would have seen a lot of smallpox, which in England in the 1700s was responsible for the deaths of thousands of children every year.

The best protection doctors could offer at the time was something called "variolation". The Chinese had realised, hundreds of years earlier, that you could protect children against the full effects of smallpox by deliberately infecting them with scabs, taken from an infected patient, which had then been left out to dry for a while.

Leaving the scabs to dry seemed to weaken the infectious agent just enough to be effective. The trick was knowing how long to leave the scabs out for. Too long and the virus would die, too short and the virus would still be extremely dangerous.

Once the scabs were ready they were ground into a fine powder which was then either blown up a child's nose or rubbed into a scratch in the skin. The child would still develop smallpox, but hopefully it would be a milder form which they were more likely to survive. Once a child had been infected they were immune for life. But it was, as you can imagine, a very hit and miss approach, as there was a serious risk of developing the full-blown disease and dying.

So there was a desperate need for something better. Then, towards the end of the 18th century, a Dorset farmer called Benjamin Jesty noticed that milkmaids who developed cowpox, unsightly pustules on their hands which came from touching the udders of infected cows, rarely got smallpox.

He was so impressed by this observation that in 1774 he rubbed scrapings taken from a milkmaid with cowpox into the arms of his wife and two children during a smallpox epidemic. They all survived.

The reason Dr Edward Jenner is remembered, and Benjamin Jesty is not, is because Jenner decided to carry out an extraordinary experiment, which these days would be regarded as completely unethical. Yet it is also an approach, which if conducted more carefully, might prove to be the fastest and most effective way of testing a new Covid-19 vaccine.

Jenner did what we would now call "a human challenge study". To prove the effectiveness of a novel vaccine you would normally give it to people at risk of getting that disease and see if it protects them when there is an outbreak. With a "human challenge study" you give your vaccine to a human volunteer, then a short while later you "challenge" that volunteer by deliberately exposing them to the virus and see if it works. Bad luck, of course, if it doesn't.

In May 1796, Jenner carried out his own version of a human challenge study. He began by infecting an eight-year-old boy called James Phipps, the son of his gardener, with pus taken from the cowpox blisters of a milkmaid called Sarah Nelmes. She in turn had caught cowpox from a cow called Blossom. After Jenner had rubbed the pus into cuts in James's forearm, the boy got a mild fever, but nothing worse.

Two months later, Jenner again scratched James's arm

and this time rubbed in pus and other "matter" taken from someone with smallpox. We don't know if either James or his family were aware of the risk that if the cowpox hadn't made him immune then James would get smallpox and might die a hideous death. If he became infectious there was also a risk that he would give smallpox to the rest of his family. Fortunately, the earlier cowpox inoculation did indeed protect him.

Jenner did the same thing to 23 other people, including his own infant son, Robert, before publishing his findings at his own expense (his paper was rejected by the Royal Society). Although he was ridiculed and savagely attacked by sceptics, including many fellow doctors, his approach was so successful it was soon being widely used. Jenner described what he was doing as "vaccination", from the Latin, *vacca*, meaning a cow.

Jenner's original experiment became so famous that when Blossom the cow, who had provided the first cowpox sample, died, her skin was preserved and hung in St George's hospital in London.

Jenner never tried to make money from his discovery. Tired of constant ridicule, he retired from public life and became a country doctor. He built a hut in his garden, which he called the "Temple of Vaccinia" and from that hut he vaccinated poor people for free. But sadly his life did not end well.

His oldest son, and his wife both died from another infectious disease, tuberculosis. He remained under constant attack by critics and shortly before dying said to a friend, "I am not surprised that men are not grateful to me; but I wonder that they are not grateful to God for the good which He has made me the instrument of conveying to my fellow creatures."

His legacy is an awesome one. What Jenner began would not only save the lives of hundreds of millions of people from smallpox, but billions more whose lives have not only been saved, but transformed by vaccination.

One irony is that modern genetic sleuths have looked at samples of smallpox vaccines, handed down the generations, and concluded that the original virus that Jenner used to inoculate young James did not actually come from a cow.

Although James Phipps was infected with pus taken from a milkmaid's hand, it seems that she may have been infected not by cowpox but by a now extinct horsepox. Jenner himself was initially convinced that what he had used was mainly horsepox. If that is right, then strictly speaking we should not be talking about "vaccination" but "equination".

The eradication of smallpox

Using Jenner's approach, a programme of successful vaccination gradually eliminated smallpox from the more affluent parts of the planet. But 140 years after Jenner's death smallpox was still killing and disfiguring more than ten million people a year. So in 1966 the WHO announced a hugely ambitious target: the complete eradication of smallpox worldwide within ten years. Donald Henderson, an American epidemiologist, was given the job.

Many eminent scientists thought the idea of global eradication was ludicrous – how could you vaccinate everyone on the planet? But Henderson had a clever plan, which avoided universal vaccination – his strategy was called Ring Vaccination.

First he ensured that there were teams of people ready to spring into action and travel to wherever there was news of a new smallpox outbreak. When they arrived at the location of the outbreak, those teams would not only vaccinate everyone in the immediate area, but also those in a larger ring around it.

The idea was that by doing this the smallpox virus would be trapped with nowhere to go and burn itself out inside the ring. The logistics, communication and co-ordination required to make such a strategy work are mind boggling – there were huge cultural and language barriers and the teams sometimes had to work in countries racked by civil war.

But village by village and country by country Henderson's team drove smallpox to the brink of extinction. In October 1977 one of his teams was sent to the Somalian port city of Merca, where they found a 23-year-old man called Ali Maow Maalin sick with smallpox.

He was immediately isolated and everyone who he had come into contact with him was tracked down and vaccinated. The team waited for more outbreaks. But there were none.

Maow Maalin was the last human to get smallpox (he survived). After thousands of years terrorising humanity, the Speckled Beast had reached the end of the line. The eradication of smallpox is one of our greatest achievements. And Henderson's strategy of Ring Vaccination could, in time, be used to contain and control future outbreaks of Covid-19.

The race for a Covid-19 vaccine begins

The good news is that 223 years on from Jenner's original experiment we have a range of safe and effective vaccines against a huge number of killer diseases, including measles, mumps, polio, cholera, tetanus, typhoid, and so on. But the bad news is that these vaccines have taken years, if not decades, to create and test. And amongst them there is no vaccine against a coronavirus.

There were attempts to make a vaccine against SARS, but these stopped when the SARS outbreak stopped. Oxford University has come closest to a successful coronavirus vaccine with one they developed against MERS, and which began human trials in Saudi Arabia in December 2019 (more on that later).

So you can see the challenge. But it is one that vaccine researchers worldwide have risen to.

The contenders

As I mentioned at the start of this chapter, there are over 100 different vaccines currently being developed and tested. Some of these vaccines are quite traditional, based on the principle of using a dead or weakened strain of the virus to alert the immune system and give it advance warning so it is better prepared when it comes face to face with the real disease.

But other groups are going down a very different route. The vaccine researchers that I've followed most closely are in the UK. One group is based at Imperial College, London, and the other at Oxford University.

Both groups believe that it is possible to produce a vaccine, in quantity, before the end of 2020. Which would be an extraordinary scientific achievement.

The Imperial approach

I first met Professor Robin Shattock, who heads the Imperial team, in his laboratory in St Mary's hospital in London. Coincidentally, St Mary's is also where, in 1928, the Scottish biologist Alexander Fleming made a remarkable discovery. While he was clearing away dishes containing cultures of bacteria called staphylococci he noticed that a mould, which had blown into his lab, had contaminated one of the dishes. Not only that, but where it had landed and was now growing it was destroying the bacteria. "That's interesting," Fleming said. It certainly was interesting because his observation would, in time, lead to the world's first safe and effective antibiotic, penicillin.

So it seems like a good omen that, nearly a century later, Robin and his team are working in the same building. Robin works in the Department of Infectious Disease at Imperial. For many years he has worked on AIDS, pioneering the use of drugs and passive antibodies to treat and prevent HIV transmission.

Robin is tall, slim and very enthusiastic. He is optimistic, such is the pace at which things are going, that by the end of the year there will be several good vaccines ready for use.

In fact one of the first things he said to me was, "With the right degree of vision and drive it really could happen. Having a vaccine to use this winter would have a major impact on reducing what we expect to be a second wave of infections. It would also help us get back on our feet again."

Robin has an unusual background for a leading academic. When he was at school he wasn't that good at science and left with poor grades. He got a job in a hospital laboratory and studied for a degree while working part time.

He was obviously a late developer because he went on to do a PhD and then spent 25 years doing pioneering research on AIDS, including novel forms of vaccine research. So he was in a great position to respond when Covid-19 reared its ugly head. To start with, like many others, he wondered if it would become a genuine threat.

"Initially we thought this was going to be a virus that comes and then goes away. We have seen a number of blips before, although we have always been aware in the scientific community that a pandemic might very well occur. But I think most of us would have predicted it would be influenza rather than a coronavirus."

It soon became clear it wasn't a blip. And then, on January 11th, 2020, Chinese scientists published the genetic sequence of the virus online. This got Robin's attention.

"The first thing we did was download that genetic sequence. Because we were very familiar with coronaviruses, we were able to rapidly utilise the genetic sequence that codes for the spikes on the surface of the virus."

The virus uses the spikes on its surface to get into human cells. With a traditional vaccine you would grow the infectious virus and then make your vaccine from killed or weakened versions of those viruses. Robin's approach is very different.

He and his team are convinced that the presence of viral spikes alone will be enough to wake up the immune system and produce an antibody response. Once your body has "learnt" to recognise that these viral spikes are foreign and need to be swamped by neutralising antibodies, it will be in a better position to rapidly respond when it encounters a real virus covered in the same spikes.

Rather than try to manufacture spikes outside the body, and then inject them, Robin wants our bodies to do the work for him, in the same way that a virus would.

To make this happen he and his team have created a vaccine made out of genetic material which is then injected into muscle. This provides the muscle cells with the genetic instructions needed to start churning out multiple copies of the viral spikes.

So, instead of doing this:

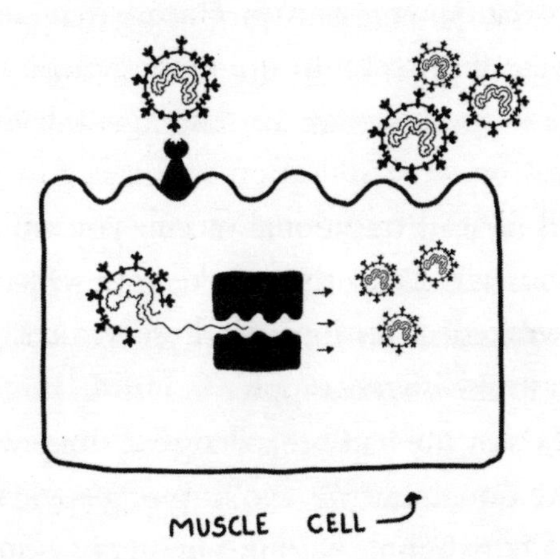

They do this:

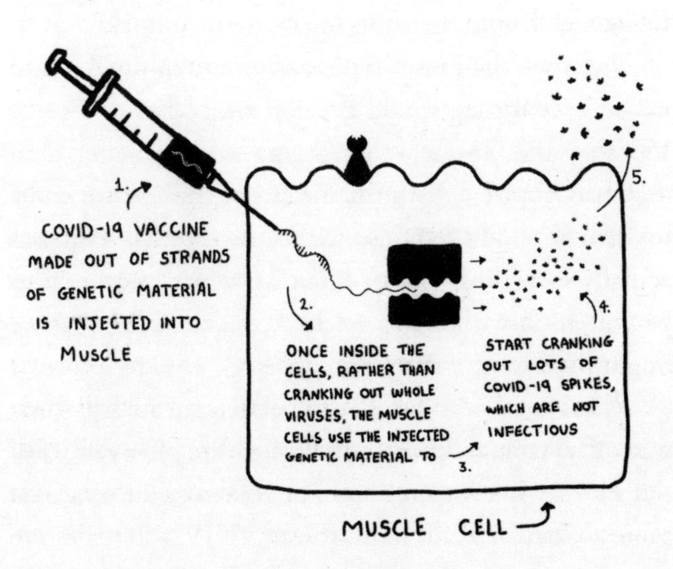

As Robin told me, "The great advantage of this approach is that you are only producing that part of the virus which will provoke an immune response. You are tricking the immune system into thinking it has seen the whole virus."

It would normally take one to two years to create a prototype vaccine. But using the data provided by the Chinese, Robin and his team were able to design their prototype vaccine on a computer in just 48 hours.

Once the vaccine had been designed, they were able to create the actual vaccine, the strip of genetic material encased in a fatty bubble, within a matter of weeks. After a few more tests, they swiftly moved on to the first real challenge. Would their vaccine work on animals?

They took their prototype vaccine and injected it into mice to see if they would develop antibodies to Covid-19. They did. In fact, the vaccine worked better than they had hoped. "With the initial experiment we saw a massive antibody response within two weeks. That was actually surprising, I don't think we were expecting it to be that good within two weeks. I was thinking that we might need to give them two doses."

This is good news but the Imperial team are still some way off a viable vaccine. Indeed, there are plenty of sceptics who say that we may never be able to create a vaccine against Covid-19 and point towards HIV, where despite more than 30 years of trying, no successful vaccine has been produced.

Having worked for many years on HIV vaccines, Robin is well aware of the challenges. But, as he pointed out, unlike AIDS, the virus that causes Covid-19 isn't mutating fast. "There is never any guarantee that things will work," he told me, "but we know that as a target this is much easier than some of the vaccines we have been trying to make because it is a relatively stable target to go after. We know we can target it with antibodies that the vaccine will induce. So we think there is a very high scientific probability that a vaccine will work."

Another major worry is whether such a radically different way of producing vaccines is likely to be safe. "That is something we will continue to monitor very carefully," he replied. "But, remember, we are not growing whole viruses and we are not using cells or animal material. The vaccine itself is a synthetic product. That is one of reasons we think the risk of side-effects is very low."

Along with genetic instructions to grow viral spikes, the Imperial vaccine contains instructions to the cell to go on making multiple copies of the spike. Which, unlike other vaccines based on this approach, makes the Imperial one self-amplifying. Which should mean you don't have to give as much. Which in turn should mean less risk of side-effects, plus you would need smaller facilities to mass-produce it.

But, of course, until you do human trials, you never know.

When I first met Robin he was frustrated because they had done all this work, on a shoe-string. They desperately needed a lot more money to take their vaccine to the next stage. I'm pleased to say that a few weeks later the health secretary announced the Imperial group were getting £22.5 million to take their work forward.

The Oxford vaccine

Another major vaccine group are based at Oxford University's Jenner Institute, named after Edward Jenner. In an interesting twist of history, although it was Alexander Fleming at St Mary's who first noticed that a penicillium mould could kill bacteria, it was scientists based in Oxford who in 1941 managed to make enough purified pencillin to treat the first human patient, a policeman called Albert Alexander.

The Oxford team are led by Sarah Gilbert, professor of vaccinology. Like the scientists at Imperial, they have created a vaccine based on targeting Covid-19's spikes, in the hope that this will induce an immune reaction that will protect people against the real thing. But their approach is very different. Their vaccine is made from a weakened version of a common cold virus (adenovirus) that causes infections in chimpanzees. It has then been genetically modified so it can't grow in humans but does produce the distinctive viral spikes of Covid-19.

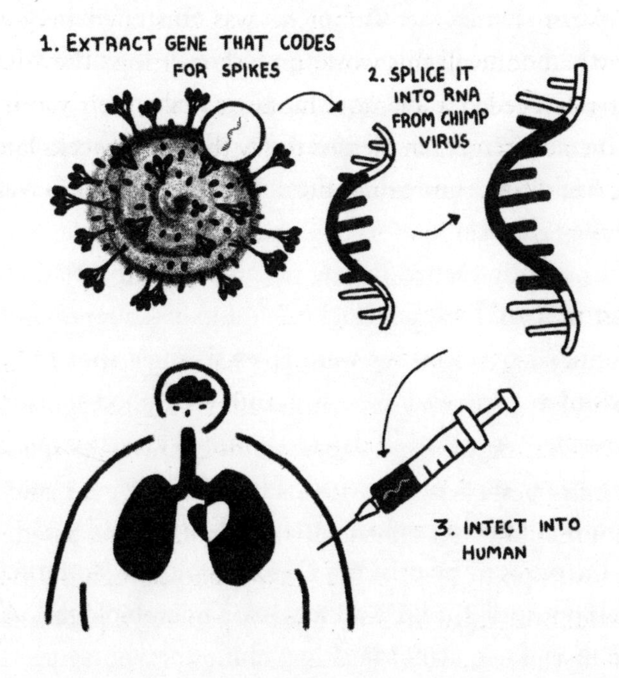

Genetically modifying a virus before injecting it may sound more complex than just injecting RNA, but unlike anyone else they have already had success using their approach on a related coronavirus.

In a study done with healthy volunteers in 2019, the Oxford group showed that their genetically modified virus was safe and could induce a good immune response against MERS. Human trials using their MERS vaccine began in Saudi Arabia in December 2019.[34]

So they were well placed when news got out that a new coronavirus, SARS-CoV-2, was on the loose. They swiftly modified their existing vaccine so it would work against Covid-19 and by March they were ready for it to be tested in macaque monkeys. Macaques are a close relative of ours and when they are infected with Covid-19 they get sick.

In a study carried out by researchers at the National Institutes of Health's Rocky Mountain Laboratory in Montana, six monkeys were given a single shot of the Oxford vaccine and they all mounted a good immune response.[35] A few weeks later, the monkeys were exposed to a heavy dose of the virus. None became sick and a month after being exposed they were still healthy.

Encouraged by this, the Oxford group began human trials on April 23rd. Elisa Granato, a microbiologist, was the first of over 1000 healthy volunteers who agreed to take part in a study where half would be given the novel vaccine, and the other half would get a control vaccine against meningitis.

Dr Granato told the BBC that she had volunteered because, "I'm a scientist, so I wanted to try to support the scientific process wherever I can."

Within days there were malicious online rumours that she and three others who had taken part in the trial, had died. "Nothing like waking up to a fake article on your death... I'm doing fine, everyone," she responded on Twitter.

So will it work? Professor Sarah Gilbert is confident it will. "I think there's a high chance that it will work, based on other things that we have done with this type of vaccine," she said, before adding that she would like to see, "tens of millions of doses manufactured before trials are complete so that if the vaccine is as safe and effective then it will be ready to distribute right away."

To make this happen the Oxford group have partnered with a huge biopharmaceutical company called AstraZeneca. They have the skills and global reach to launch into large-scale manufacture and distribution of a Covid-19 vaccine as soon as one comes available.

Oxford want the vaccine to be as widely used as possible, so they have also lined up seven other companies to begin manufacturing the vaccine. Three of them in the UK, two in Europe, one in India and one in China.

Other potential vaccines

A number of other vaccine makers have also begun

human trials. One of the most promising is an American company called Moderna, who have teamed up with the Vaccine Research Center at the National Institutes of Health in the US. Like the Imperial vaccine, their approach is based on injecting the genetic instructions to build viral spikes into humans and hoping that will provoke an immune response

They were very fast out of the blocks and did their first test on a human volunteer on March 15th, as part of a "Phase I" study, where they were assessing safety and whether people mount an antibody response.

On May 7th they got approval from the US Food and Drug Administration (FDA) to begin "Phase II" human trials (again, mainly to assess safety and how well people respond), involving around 600 volunteers. If that trial goes well, they are hoping to go into Phase III trials (where they test just how effective it really is) this summer.

A more traditional approach

Not all the vaccines being tested are high-tech. Sinovac, a company based in Beijing, have made a vaccine, using a much more traditional approach. They began by collecting samples of Covid-19 viruses from infected patients, which they then purified and inactivated. In 2003 Sinovac used this approach to create a vaccine against SARS, and even began using it in early human trials. But the vaccine wasn't taken any further because the SARS outbreak ended, so there was no way of testing its real effectiveness. They are hoping for better luck with this one.

In March 2020, like the Oxford group, they first injected monkeys with their vaccine. Three weeks later they did a "challenge" experiment, exposing the monkeys to the Covid-19 virus. The vaccine seemed to protect them, because unlike the control group (who didn't get the vaccine) none of the vaccinated group became ill.

In April they started human trials with 144 healthy volunteers.

Potential problems

This all sounds remarkably positive, so what could go wrong? Well, there are plenty of sceptics who think that creating a safe and effective vaccine against Covid-19 will take years, or even decades. These are some of their arguments.

People who have been infected with Covid-19 are getting infected again.

There were reports from South Korea that some people

who had tested positive for the virus had gone down with the disease for a second time, which would suggest that some people don't develop proper immunity. But it now appears that cases of "re-infection" were actually because of faulty testing.

It turns out that the repeat tests, which detected viral genetic material in people who had previously been ill, were actually detecting dead virus fragments which can remain in the body for weeks, possibly for months. There was no evidence of active virus.

Further encouraging research comes from studies done with monkeys, who have been deliberately infected with the Covid-19 virus, recovered, and then exposed to the virus again. All the monkeys mounted a good response and none got infected the second time round.

Even if we develop immunity, it won't last

One of the main fears is that, even if a vaccine works, the impact won't last. Although it may not give you lifelong immunity (which the smallpox vaccine does), there are good reasons to hope the effects of a vaccine will last at least a year.

A Chinese study, looking at 176 people who got SARS, which is caused by a related coronavirus, found that they maintained good levels of antibody against the virus for a couple of years, and some for up to 14 years.[36]

It is true that some of the people they tested did have low levels of antibody after less than two years, but that doesn't mean that they wouldn't be protected if they were exposed again. The worst it suggests is that some people may need a booster shot.

A vaccine could make the disease worse

With some experimental vaccines there has been a phenomenon called "disease enhancement", where those who've been vaccinated become sicker when exposed to the virus than people who've not been vaccinated. It happened in 1966 when a few children, who had been given an experimental vaccine for RSV, a common respiratory virus, developed more severe disease.

The reason people fear this could happen with a Covid-19 is because of a trial in 2004 of an experimental SARS vaccine. Development of the vaccine was stopped when the animals who'd been vaccinated (in this case, ferrets) developed serious liver disease after being infected with the SARS virus.

So far none of the Covid-19 vaccine researchers I've spoken to have seen disease enhancement in any of the animals they've treated. The reason researchers do extensive studies with healthy volunteers is to pick up potential side-effects. But until those human volunteers get exposed to the virus you can't be absolutely certain it is completely safe, or that it works.

You may be able to produce a vaccine in the next few months, but it will take years to test

In normal times creating a safe and effective vaccine takes at least five years because they have to go through rigorous testing and lots of regulatory hoops. 95% of potential vaccines fail. The steps a normal vaccine has to go through include:

- Step one: exploratory stage

This is when you do your basic lab research and create your vaccine. This often takes two to four years.

- Pre-clinical stage

This is when you do things like animal testing, to see if your vaccine is safe and produces a suitable response. It usually takes another couple of years and most vaccines fail at this stage.

- Phase I trials

Once you feel sure it works in animals, you move on to testing it on a small group of healthy adults. Is the vaccine safe and does it provoke a good immune response in humans?

• Phase II trials

Assuming your vaccine passes Phase I, you move on to a bigger trial, involving several hundred volunteers. In these trials the volunteers are randomised to either getting the vaccine, or a harmless placebo. Again, what you are trying to assess is how safe the vaccine is, how good it is at arousing the immune system and what sort of dose you should be giving.

• Phase III trials

If your vaccine gets this far then it will be tested on thousands or tens of thousands of people. With phase III trials, people are again randomised to getting the vaccine or a placebo. This is when you find out if the people who've had the vaccine are better protected against getting the disease, or get it more mildly, than those who were given the placebo.

Doing Phase III trials the traditional way, with Covid-19, could be tricky. To find out if your vaccine works, the people you vaccinate then have to be exposed to the disease. But if you have successfully crushed the curve and there is not a lot of Covid-19 in circulation, you may have to hang around for the next wave to see if your vaccine is effective.

As Professor Adrian Hill, the Jenner Institute's director, told *The New York Times* in April, "We're the only people in the country who want the number of new infections to stay up for another few weeks, so we can test our vaccine."[37]

There are alternatives. You could do your Phase III vaccine trials in a country where the disease is still very active. Or you could do a human challenge test, like Dr Edward Jenner did, all those years ago. That would involve vaccinating healthy individuals and then deliberately exposing them to Covid-19 to see if it protected them. But would that be ethical?

The challenge of human challenge experiments

The argument against doing a human challenge experiment is that you are asking people to expose themselves to the risk of serious disease or even death if something goes wrong. A recent article written by experts from Harvard and the London School of Hygiene and Tropical Medicine argue that it can be justified.[38]

They point out that a human challenge experiment, by speeding up development of a vaccine, could save many lives. "Every week that vaccine roll-out is delayed will be accompanied by many thousands of deaths globally," they write. "If the use of human challenge helped to make the vaccine available before the epidemic has completely passed, the savings in human lives could be in the thousands or conceivably millions."

To minimise the risk to volunteers, they would have to be young and healthy, so you know that they are at low risk of complications if they get Covid-19.

You would also need to ensure that they are closely monitored and get the best possible care if something goes wrong. Ideally you would have drugs to hand that would help. Drugs which don't currently exist, or at least are unproven.

Finally you could recruit your volunteers from a group who are likely to get exposed to the virus anyway, such as frontline workers. We already expect frontline medical staff to risk themselves by treating patients with Covid-19. Is this really that different?

When I was a medical student I took part in a couple of studies of new drugs, where they needed healthy volunteers to test for potential side-effects. If I was the right age (I am, sadly, too old), I wouldn't hesitate to volunteer.

A website, 1 Day Sooner (https://1daysooner.org), has been created, looking for potential volunteers. It was set up by Josh Morrison, a corporate lawyer who donated his kidney to a stranger in 2011. As he pointed out in a recent newspaper article, "We and many others are willing to take on what we see as an acceptable individual risk to serve the public and the people we care about. As willing and well-informed volunteers, whose autonomy ought to be respected, we feel challenge trials are justified if they mean a vaccine arrives even one day sooner."[39]

They point out that, if you are a healthy 20-29-year-old, then even if you get Covid-19 your risk of dying is roughly the same as donating a kidney or having an appendix removed.

It seems there are plenty of people out there prepared to take the risk for the greater good. When I last looked the website had clocked up more than 15,000 potential volunteers from over 100 countries.

The WHO also thinks human challenge studies are acceptable. On May 6th they published guidelines, including eight criteria which must be met before such studies can go ahead.[40]

6 The future

There is hope, but one of the things I find hard to accept, emotionally, is that we are just at the start of this crisis. In many countries death rates are falling, but in others they are beginning to rise. Countries like New Zealand and Australia have managed to control the virus by cutting themselves off from the rest of the world, but it is hard to see others doing so, long term.

Until we get a vaccine, we are going to have to find ways to live with this virus. One approach, for the countries who can afford it, will be to follow the example of South Korea.

That means social distancing, wearing masks in public, lots of testing and extensive tracking. Widespread testing, along with tracking, means that people who've been infected can be detected, isolated and treated before they spread it to others.

But doing it the South Korean way involves major privacy issues. In South Korea an emergency law means officials can trace your movements by using surveillance cameras and accessing data from your phone. If you've crossed paths with someone who has recently tested positive, you're sent a text and told to report to a testing centre. If you test positive, you're sent to a government shelter or told to go home, depending on your circumstances. If you test negative, you still have to self-isolate and download an app which tells the police if you go outside. You can be fined or sent to jail for failing to comply.

Some countries, like the UK, are trialling the voluntary use of tracker apps, to let people know when they have been exposed to the virus. But experts say that to be effective at least 60% of the population would need to download and use the app.[41] Will enough people do that voluntarily?

Now there are reliable antibody tests we may also get the widespread use of immunity passports. These would be digital documents, probably stored on your phone, which prove that you have been infected and that you are now immune. People with immunity passports would be allowed to return to work and a relatively normal daily life. But immunity passports would be open to fraud and some people, who test negative, might be tempted to try and get infected so that they can get an immunity passport.

Going forwards, we will almost certainly have to use a "lift, supress, lift" approach to social distancing. Children will go back to school, universities will open and restrictions on social gatherings will be relaxed. But as soon as there are signs that the virus is spreading again, on will go the brakes. The continuing uncertainty will be hugely damaging to large parts of the economy.

Along with damage to the economy there is likely to be a second wave, not just more infections but more mental illness. During the last recession, from 2007-2009, the rise in unemployment led to a spike in suicide rates in the United States and Europe, up by more than 10,000 people.[42]

Hugs, handshakes, and large social gatherings are off the menu for the foreseeable future. People are already becoming intensely anxious about going outside and mixing with others. What will happen to elderly people, like my mother? How can we keep them safe without keeping them physically isolated?

On the plus side, I hope people will continue to wash their hands, which could dramatically cut the risk of another major flu outbreak. I expect we will fly less, travel less and work more from home. We will be more appreciative of our healthcare workers and people who work in social care. This crisis may, paradoxically, make us more communal.

It may even make us care more about the state of the planet, put pressure on politicians to stamp out the illegal trade in endangered species, which have played such a big part in the current crisis.

It is going to be a long, hard road back to any form of normality. But if you are an optimist, which I am, you have to hope that this pandemic will bring out the best in us and bring the world together to deal more effectively with future global challenges.

Endnotes

1 https://www.nature.com/articles/s41586-020-2196-x
2 https://www.ncbi.nlm.nih.gov/books/NBK143281/
3 https://www.medrxiv.org/content/10.1101/2020.03.09.20033217v1.full.pdf
4 https://dontforgetthebubbles.com/evidence-summary-paediatric-covid-19-literature/
5 https://www.cebm.net/covid-19/global-covid-19-case-fatality-rates/
6 https://www.nytimes.com/2020/04/27/health/coronavirus-estrogen-men.html
7 https://www.icnarc.org/Our-Audit/Audits/Cmp/Reports
8 https://www.ons.gov.uk/peoplepopulationandcommunity/birthsdeathsandmarriages/deaths/articles/coronavirusrelateddeathsbyethnicgroupenglandandwales/2march2020to10april2020
9 https://www.thelancet.com/journals/lancet/article/PIIS0140-6736(20)30183-5/fulltext#bib35
10 https://www.scientificamerican.com/article/how-chinas-bat-woman-hunted-down-viruses-from-sars-to-the-new-coronavirus1/
11 https://www.nytimes.com/2020/02/01/world/asia/china-coronavirus.html
12 https://www.medrxiv.org/content/10.1101/2020.02.04.20020479v2
13 https://www.who.int/csr/don/12-january-2020-novel-coronavirus-china/en/
14 https://apnews.com/68a9e1b91de4ffc166acd6012d82c2f9
15 https://www.thelancet.com/journals/lancet/article/PIIS0140-6736(20)30154-9/fulltext
16 https://www.nytimes.com/2020/04/04/us/coronavirus-china-travel-restrictions.html

17 https://www.imperial.ac.uk/media/imperial-college/medicine/sph/ide/gida-fellowships/Imperial-College-COVID19-NPI-modelling-16-03-2020.pdf
18 https://www.imperial.ac.uk/news/196496/coronavirus-pandemic-could-have-caused-40/
19 https://www.insidescience.org/news/how-viruses-secretly-control-planet
20 https://www.nytimes.com/2016/03/03/science/study-finds-surprising-benefit-of-viral-dna-fighting-other-viruses.html?action=click&module=RelatedCoverage&pgtype=Article®ion=Footer
21 https://wwwnc.cdc.gov/eid/article/26/7/20-0764_article
22 https://wwwnc.cdc.gov/eid/article/26/8/20-1274_article
23 https://news.yahoo.com/sunlight-destroys-coronavirus-very-quickly-new-government-tests-find-but-experts-say-pandemic-could-still-last-through-summer-200745675.html?guccounter=1
24 https://www.fast.ai/2020/04/13/masks-summary/
25 https://www.niaid.nih.gov/news-events/nih-clinical-trial-shows-remdesivir-accelerates-recovery-advanced-covid-19
26 https://www.medrxiv.org/content/10.1101/2020.04.16.20065920v1.full.pdf
27 https://www.health.harvard.edu/diseases-and-conditions/flu-vaccine-less-effective-in-obese-individuals
28 https://www.directclinicaltrial.org.uk/
29 https://bmjopen.bmj.com/content/7/8/e016709
30 https://www.phc.ox.ac.uk/research/participate/diamond
31 https://www.frontiersin.org/articles/10.3389/fphys.2018.00997/full
32 https://www.ncbi.nlm.nih.gov/pubmed/26118561
33 https://www.sciencedirect.com/science/article/abs/pii/S0889159116305645?via%3Dihub
34 http://www.ox.ac.uk/news/2019-12-19-new-mers-vaccine-clinical-trial-starts-saudi-arabia

35 https://www.nytimes.com/2020/04/27/world/europe/coronavirus-vaccine-update-oxford.html

36 https://www.ncbi.nlm.nih.gov/pmc/articles/PMC2851497/

37 https://www.nytimes.com/2020/04/27/world/europe/coronavirus-vaccine-update-oxford.html

38 https://academic.oup.com/jid/advance-article/doi/10.1093/infdis/jiaa152/5814216

39 https://www.nytimes.com/2020/04/30/opinion/coronavirus-vaccine-covid.html

40 https://apps.who.int/iris/bitstream/handle/10665/331976/WHO-2019-nCoV-Ethics_criteria-2020.1-eng.pdf?ua=1

41 https://www.bdi.ox.ac.uk/news/digital-contact-tracing-can-slow-or-even-stop-coronavirus-transmission-and-ease-us-out-of-lockdown

42 https://www.reuters.com/investigates/special-report/health-coronavirus-usa-cost/

Dr Michael Mosley is a science presenter, journalist and executive producer. After training to be a doctor at the Royal Free Hospital in London, he spent 25 years at the BBC, where he made numerous science documentaries. Now freelance, he is the author of several bestselling books, *The Fast Diet*, *The 8-Week Blood Sugar Diet*, *The Clever Guts Diet, The Fast 800* and *Fast Asleep*. He is married with four children.